To John Crossley
with thanks from
Joe Sage

Joseph

PEDIATRIC AND ADOLESCENT ECHOCARDIOGRAPHY

Pediatric and Adolescent Echocardiography

A Handbook

STANLEY J. GOLDBERG, M.D., *Professor*
HUGH D. ALLEN, M.D., *Assistant Professor*
DAVID J. SAHN, M.D., *Assistant Professor*

Department of Pediatrics
Cardiology
The University of Arizona College of Medicine

YEAR BOOK MEDICAL PUBLISHERS, INC.
35 East Wacker Drive • Chicago

Library of Congress Catalog Card Number: 74-18153
International Standard Book Number: 0-8151-3719-2

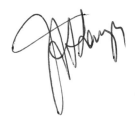

To our wives and children

Elaine, Susan, Steven and Mark Goldberg
Elizabeth, Clark and Carl Allen
Beverly and Jennifer Sahn

Preface

A BRITISH SERGEANT is purported to have told his troops during a map-reading orientation that whenever a discrepancy exists between the map and the ground, the ground usually is correct.

Echocardiography is a rapidly emerging noninvasive diagnostic tool that will become indispensable for complete evaluation of children with congenital cardiac disease.

Accurate observation of a properly performed study is essential for correct interpretation. In echocardiography, the ground and the map are correct, but the latter can be technically distorted by the echocardiographer. Failure to recognize this induced distortion is the major hazard of echocardiography.

The scope of this book will be greater than congenital disease, as echocardiographic principles, as well as specific diseases, will be emphasized. It thus will be useful to the cardiologist (pediatrician or internist), house officer and student. Knowledge of some basic cardiologic concepts will be assumed at the level taught to medical students. This book will teach the reader to critically examine the echocardiogram, differentiate normal from abnormal and emphasize pitfalls in interpretation and technique. In this text we will relate our observations to those of others. Comprehensive referencing will be provided. Collective knowledge of the scope of normal and range of abnormal is presented. A self-assessment section is the main feature of Chapter 6. The final chapter is devoted to early results of cross-sectional echographic studies.

ACKNOWLEDGMENTS

General Acknowledgments

Our first very important acknowledgment goes to Marla Gillham for typing, coordinating and strokes of genius during the preparation of the manuscript. To our medical art and photography department, specifically Mr. Cliff Pollack, Mr. James Coons and Mr. Mark Pederson, for providing outstanding illustrations, photography and a great deal of cooperation. To our echocardiographers, Mrs. Iris Wright, Ms. Wendy George, Ms. Nancy Schy and Ms. Janice Wood, for performing many of the echocardiograms included in the text. To Dr. Vincent A. Fulginiti, our pediatrics departmental chairman, for providing us the environment in which to accomplish the task. To Dr. Frank Marcus for allowing us to develop echocardiography early and rapidly at The University of Arizona. To the physicians of Tucson and Arizona, who provided us patient material, and to Drs. Mark Herman and John Carr, directors of Crippled Children's Services and State Health Department, State of Nevada, for rapidly developing echocardiography in The University of Arizona—Las Vegas, Nevada Crippled Children's Services Clinic. Many of the echocardiograms in this text are from this source.

Individual Acknowledgments

STANLEY J. GOLDBERG

First, I would like to acknowledge the individual who has contributed most to my echocardiographic education, Dr. Harvey Feigenbaum, both by his personal instruction and his excellent research and publications. Also, I would like to acknowledge the echocardiographic educational assistance of Sonia Chang and Dr. Lee Konecke. Finally, I wish to acknowledge those who contributed most to my pediatric cardiac education, Drs. Jerome Liebman, Leonard Linde and Victor Hall.

HUGH D. ALLEN

I would like to acknowledge Drs. Russell V. Lucas, Jr., James H. Moller, Ray C. Anderson, Leonard C. Blieden and Howard B. Burchell of the University of Minnesota for encouragement, support and criticism during my embryonic echo experience. I would also like to acknowledge Drs. Richard Meyer and Samuel Kaplan of the University of Cincinnati for early instruction and continued support with my echocardiographic endeavors.

DAVID J. SAHN

The multicrystal cross-sectional echocardiographic techniques presented herein were performed with a prototype instrument designed by Dr. Klaas Bom, Chief of Section on Experimental Echocardiography, Erasmus University, Rotterdam, The Netherlands, and supplied by Organon Teknika, B. V. Oss, The Netherlands. Studies were performed under the supervision and guidance of Dr. William F. Friedman, Chief of Pediatric Cardiology, University of California—San Diego, who was instrumental in this application of cross-sectional echocardiographic methods to pediatric patients. Appreciation is expressed to Drs. George Leopold, Robert O'Rourke, Arthur

Hagan and Richard Popp and to Susan Shackleton and Sandra Hagan for instruction, support, encouragement, cooperation and patience during the acquisition of the cross-sectional and newborn echo data.

Contents

Common Echocardiographic Abbreviations

Abbreviation	Translation
AAC	Anterior Aortic Cusp
AAO	Ascending Aorta
AAW	Anterior Aortic Wall
AM	Anterior Mitral Valve Leaflet
AML	Anterior Mitral Valve Leaflet
AMVL	Anterior Mitral Valve Leaflet
AO	Aorta
AO ARCH	Aortic Arch
AO D	Aortic Dimension
ARVW	Anterior Right Ventricular Wall
ASCENDING AO	Ascending Aorta
ASH	Asymmetric Septal Hypertrophy
ATL	Anterior Tricuspid Leaflet
AV	Aortic Valve
C	Chordae, Catheter
CL	Common Leaflet (Endocardial Cushion Defect)
CW	Chest Wall
D	Dye – indocyanine for contrast studies
Dd	Diastolic Dimension
defabc	Points and Slopes of Mitral and Tricuspid Valve Motion
Ds	Systolic Dimension
e	Endocardium
ECG	Electrocardiogram
en	Endocardium
EP	Epicardium
epi	Epicardium
IcD	Intercusp Distance

Abbreviation	Translation
IVS	Interventricular Septum
LA	Left Atrium
LAA	Left Atrial Appendage
LA-AO	Left Atrium-Aorta
LAD	Left Atrial Dimension
LAID	Left Atrial Internal Dimension
LAPW	Left Atrial Posterior Wall
LS	Left Septal Surface
LV	Left Ventricle
LVD	Left Ventricular Dimension
LVID	Left Ventricular Internal Dimension
$LVID_d$	Left Ventricular Internal Dimension, Diastolic
$LVID_s$	Left Ventricular Internal Dimension, Systolic
LVPW	Left Ventricular Posterior Wall
MPA	Main Pulmonary Artery
MS	Membranous Septum
MV	Mitral Valve
MYO	Myocardium
P	Papillary Muscle, Pericardium
PA	Pulmonary Artery
PAC	Posterior Aortic Cusp
PAW	Posterior Aortic Wall
Per	Pericardium

1

PLA	Posterior Left Atrial Wall	RVID	Right Ventricular Internal Dimension
PM	Papillary Muscle (Anterior), Posterior Mitral Leaflet	RVOT	Right Ventricular Outflow Tract
PML	Posterior Mitral Leaflet	RVW	Right Ventricular Anterior Wall
PMVL	Posterior Mitral Valve Leaflet	S	Septum
PPM	Posterior Papillary Muscle	SAM	Systolic Anterior Motion
PPV	Posterior Pulmonary Valve Leaflet	SD	Septal Depth
		Sept	Septum
PUL	Pulmonary Artery	SSN	Suprasternal Notch
PV	Pulmonary Valve	SV	Single Ventricle, Stroke Volume
PVOD	Pulmonary Vascular Obstructive Disease	SVAS	Supravalvular Aortic Stenosis
		TA	Tricuspid Annulus
RA	Right Atrium	Tri	Tricuspid Valve
RPA	Right Pulmonary Artery	TV	Tricuspid Valve
		Vcf	Velocity of Circumferential Fiber Shortening
RSS	Right Septal Surface		
RV	Right Ventricle	Y AXIS	Superior-Inferior Axis
RVAW	Right Ventricular Anterior Wall	Y LAD	Superior-Inferior Axis Left Atrial Dimension
RVC	Right Ventricular Cavity		
RV CAV	Right Ventricular Cavity	Z AXIS	Anteroposterior Axis
RVD	Right Ventricular Dimension	Z LAD	Anteroposterior Axis Left Atrial Dimension

1 / An Introduction to the Physics of Ultrasound

THE PHYSICS OF ULTRASOUND is a complex and vast subject. No attempt will be made to review this subject comprehensively. The reader interested in more detail is referred to volumes that cover this material in depth.[86, 104, 123, 232] However, a few basic concepts are necessary for the physician or technician who wishes to understand echocardiography.

FREQUENCY

In order to understand the physics of ultrasound, one first must understand frequency. Frequency is defined as the number of events that occur in one unit of time. The basic event with respect to sound is a cycle of compression and expansion. As sound passes through a substance, the particles of that substance are alternately compressed and expanded. Each particle passes the motion on to its adjacent particle, thus passing a wave through the substance. Since one expansion and one compression represent one cycle, the total number of cycles per second is termed frequency. Until a few years ago, the unit of frequency was designated as the cycle per second (cps), but recently it was renamed "the Hertz" (Hz). One Hz is equal to one cycle per second.

A normal ear can perceive sound frequencies as low as 30–50 Hz and as high as 15,000 Hz. Ultrasound is defined as sound of a frequency greater than 20,000 Hz.[232] Medical diagnostic work requires frequencies in the range of millions of Hz.

WAVELENGTH

Wavelength is defined as the linear distance between successive wave fronts. Since the wave fronts are all traveling at the same speed, the distance between successive wave fronts is inversely related to the frequency with which they are generated; i.e., wave fronts generated at higher frequency have less distance between them and therefore a shorter wavelength.

VELOCITY

Velocity is the speed at which sound travels through a medium. It is a function of the density and elastic properties of the medium.

3

Frequency (f), wavelength (λ) and velocity (v) are related according to the equation $v = f \times \lambda$; i.e., velocity is a function of frequency times wavelength.

Since velocity is also a function of the medium through which the sound travels, the velocity of ultrasound through body tissue is an important factor in diagnostic work. If the time required for the sound waves to pass through a part of the body is known, and if that part acts as a uniform conductor of sound, the distance that the sound has traveled can be computed. Velocity (cm/sec) × Time (sec) = Distance (cm).

Fortunately, the body generally resembles a uniform conductor and sound travels through it at about 1540 meters per second.[83, 86, 137] This is an oversimplification, for the velocity in bone is more than twice as fast as the velocity in soft tissue, and the velocity in air is much slower. Average velocities are as follows[83, 137]:

MEDIUM	ACTUAL VELOCITY	VELOCITY ASSUMED
Saline	1534 m/sec	1540 m/sec
Soft tissue	1540 m/sec	1540 m/sec
Bone	3380 m/sec	1540 m/sec
Air @ 37°C	354 m/sec	350 m/sec ·

For cardiac work, the approximation of 1540 m/sec is reasonable, since it is difficult to penetrate the sternum and ribs with sufficient ultrasound for diagnostic work and air-bearing structures stop sound penetration. Accordingly, in the adult and older child, echocardiograms usually are performed through the interspaces between the third and fourth ribs. In infants, it usually is possible to pass sufficient ultrasound through the cartilaginous rib cage and sternum to get a diagnostic tracing, probably because these structures still are quite thin and may not be completely ossified. Any velocity error introduced by transmitting sound through bone in infants is small and usually can be ignored.

ACOUSTIC IMPEDANCE

Acoustic impedance is the density of a medium times the velocity with which sound passes through that medium. When an interface (boundary between two media) of two materials of different acoustic impedance is encountered by a beam of ultrasound, some of the ultrasound will be reflected from that interface and some will pass through it into the second material. The amount of ultrasound that is reflected is determined by the formula

$$\text{Reflection index} = \frac{\rho_1 v_1 - \rho_2 v_2}{\rho_1 v_1 + \rho_2 v_2}$$

where ρ_1 and ρ_2 are the respective densities and v_1 and v_2 are the respective velocities through the medium.

The greater the difference in acoustic impedance the greater will be the energy reflected at any given angle of incidence. The beam may strike an interface at any angle, and the more perpendicular the beam is to the interface the greater will be the amount of returned sound reflection. Additionally, if the interface is intercepted at the perpendicular by the beam, the reflected wave will return to the source. On the other hand, if the beam strikes at an angle that varies from the perpendicular to the interface, the reflected wave will not return to the source but be angled away from it. This principle is similar to that of throwing a ball against a wall. If the ball is thrown so that it travels at a perpendicular to the wall, it will return to the thrower. If the ball strikes the wall at an angle of 45°, it will reflect off the wall at 45° and not return to the thrower. This concept is important in ultrasound work, for even though the beam may strike the desired structure, if it does so at an angle other than one near the perpendicular, the reflected wave will not be sensed at the site at which it was generated.

TRANSDUCERS

Some knowledge of transducers is fundamental to diagnostic ultrasound. A transducer is a device that can sense an event and transform it into an electrical signal. Transducers used in ultrasound have an additional aspect—they also create sound. The piezoelectric ("pressure-electric") effect is the ability of a substance to transform a mechanical strain into an electrical charge and vice versa. A number of crystalline substances found in nature have this property. If a small plate of crystal that possesses the property is placed between two conducting electrodes, it will be mechanically deformed when the electrodes are connected to a source of voltage. Conversely, if the crystal between two electrodes is deformed by pressure, a voltage will be developed between the electrodes. Piezoelectric devices are encountered most commonly in microphones and phonograph cartridges, where mechanical vibrations are transformed into alternating voltages of corresponding frequency. The reverse capability is used commonly in headphones and loudspeakers, where electrical energy is transformed into mechanical vibrations that are recognized as sound.

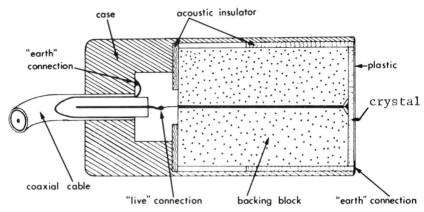

Fig. 1-1. – Construction of an ultrasonic transducer. (Modified after P.N.T. Wells, *Physical Principles of Ultrasonic Diagnosis* [London and New York: Academic Press, 1969].)

These crystalline plates are also mechanical resonators that have natural frequencies of vibration ranging from a few thousand Hz to tens of megahertz (MHz). The vibrating frequency depends on the type of crystal, the way the plate was cut from the natural crystal and the dimension of the plate.

Ceramic substances are used as the piezoelectric element in ultrasonic transducers. A backing material absorbs energy directed toward it and also affects the transmission of forward energy (Fig. 1-1). The piezoelectric effect is shown diagrammatically in Figure 1-2. In panel A, the piezoelectric crystal has widely separated particles. In panel B, the crystal is compressed by an electrical signal from the echocardiograph and sound waves are generated. Panel C shows restoration of the crystal. The sound waves continue their path and strike two reflecting surfaces, "x" and "y." Since "x" is perpendicular to the wave front, the reflected waves return toward the crystal. Reflections from surface "y" are not returned to the crystal. In panel D, the reflected waves from "x" compress the crystal and an electrical signal is sent back to the echograph. The echoscope display shows two echoes, one representing the transducer interface with the system and the second representing the returning echoes from surface "x."

DIVERGENCE

It would be ideal if the ultrasound transducer produced only a constant narrow beam of sound, but this is not the case. The unfo-

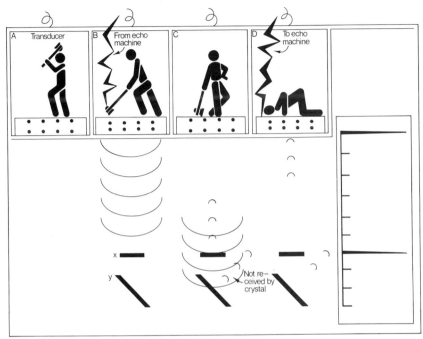

Fig. 1-2.—The piezoelectric effect and diagrammatic representation of sound reflection. The details are covered in the text. The transducer state is depicted in panels $A-D$. Particle compression and expansion are represented by the vertical distance between particles in each panel. Panels A and C depict the crystal at rest. Panels B and D show compression of the particles by an electric signal (B) and by reflected sound, which creates an electric signal (D). It should be obvious, but is not shown, that B and D are not only compressed but also expand cyclically at the frequency of the transducer. At rest, as shown in panels A and C, no compression or expansion is occurring. The small echoes are used to diagrammatically represent reflection and are shown at the same frequency as the larger incident echoes. At the far right is the face of an echoscope with an A-mode display. This display is discussed in detail in Chapter 2. Two echoes are produced, one at the transducer interface and another at the X plate, since signals return from that surface to the transducer. As the echoscope shows reflected echoes, the presence of the plate is confirmed. For purposes of this diagram, the echoscope is shown to be exactly calibrated with respect to the distance between the transducer and plate X.

cused beam maintains this ideal character for a certain distance, the near field. Then the beam begins to widen in the far field (Fig. 1-3). The point at which divergence occurs may be computed according to the formula $d = r^2/\lambda$, where d is the distance to the far field, r is the

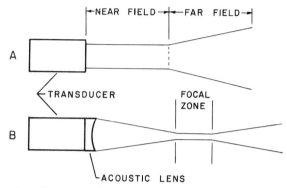

Fig. 1-3.—Transducers with and without acoustic lenses are shown diagrammatically. In **A**, the beam is columnar (the near field) and then diverges (the far field). In **B**, an acoustic lens is used to create a focal zone beyond the far field that would have existed if no lens were used. However, the focal zone is relatively short and then divergence occurs again.

transducer radius and λ is the wavelength of the transducer. The near field of more commonly used transducers is:

Diameter	Frequency	Wavelength	Near Field
$\frac{1}{2}''$ (r = 6 mm)	2.5 MHz	0.6 mm	60 mm
$\frac{1}{4}''$ (r = 3 mm)	2.5 MHz	0.6 mm	15 mm
$\frac{1}{4}''$ (r = 3 mm)	5.0 MHz	0.3 mm	30 mm
$\frac{1}{4}''$ (r = 3 mm)	7.5 MHz	0.2 mm	45 mm

The divergence after the near field can be computed from the formula $\sin \alpha = 0.61 \, \lambda/r$, where α = the angle of divergence.[46, 232]

To overcome divergence, acoustic "lenses" have been added to create a focal zone and decrease divergence (Fig. 1-3, *B*). Transducers with acoustic lenses have been helpful in adult patients and in older children with hearts deep in relation to the anterior chest wall, but we have not found them to be necessary for most children. The reason for this probably is that most cardiac structures in children occur at a depth of 20–60 mm from the transducer. This places the structures either in the near field or at a point of only slight divergence. In the adult, cardiac structures are located much farther from the transducer. Therefore, the problem of divergence is more important in the adult.

DEPTH RESOLUTION

Resolution refers to the ability to differentiate and recognize the separation of structures that are physically close to one another. The physician probably is most accustomed to thinking of resolution in terms of the number of lines per inch that can be resolved on an x-ray. Ultrasonic resolution is similar in concept. The thickness of a structure must be at least one-fourth of an ultrasonic wavelength before it can be recognized as a separate entity.[232] Since the wavelength of ultrasound at 2.5 MHz is 0.6 mm and at 7.5 MHz is 0.2 mm, a 2.5-MHz transducer could resolve structures as close as 0.15 mm and a 7.5-MHz transducer could resolve structures 0.05 mm apart. However, a price is paid for the increased resolution at high frequencies, for many surfaces are encountered that reflect or absorb the ultrasound. Therefore, less sound is available for further penetration. A general principle can be stated. As frequencies increase, greater resolution is attained but less sound penetration is possible. Sound is "used up." This information can be used when transducers are selected for a given task. An adult patient would require a low-frequency transducer in order to obtain the necessary penetration of ultrasound. On the other hand, a premature infant whose cardiac posterior wall is 2–3 cm from the transducer and who has very small cardiac structures should be examined with a high-frequency transducer. As a general rule, in the premature, low-frequency transducers result in very poor resolution, and accurate diagnosis is more difficult.

TRANSMITTER-RECEIVER

It is useful to think of the echocardiograph as a transmitter and receiver of sound. The transmitted sound is created by providing electrical energy to the transducer crystal. This sets up the previously described contractions and expansions at the natural frequency of the crystal, and these vibrations result in the creation of ultrasound. The echocardiograph transmits sound part of the time, then ceases transmission and "listens" for reflected sound during the remainder of the cycle. The portion of the cycle that is devoted to transmitting and receiving varies from manufacturer to manufacturer, but usually has a ratio of more than 99 to 1 in favor of receiving. The number of these transmitting-receiving cycles that occur depends on the instrument, but most commonly is 1000/sec. This is called "pulsing" and is also referred to as a repetition or sampling rate. Thus, an event that occurs in 1 msec can be recognized, but an event that occurs in less than 1 msec could be missed. In diagnostic cardiac work, this is insignificant because no observable biologic cardiac events occur that fast. The number of transmitted pulses per second is referred to as "repetition" or "sampling rate." This is not to be confused with the frequency of the transducer, which is a function of the physical characteristics of the crystal in the transducer.

DISPLAY

Figure 1-4 is useful in helping to understand the ultrasound display. The transducer is attached to a cylinder *(A–C)*, which has a plate at point *B*. If the cylinder is filled with air, no significant amount of ultrasound can be passed through it, for air is a very poor conductor of ultrasound. If the cylinder is filled with a fluid, such as saline, ultrasound will pass from the transducer through the saline to plate *B* with a velocity of 1534 m/sec. Some ultrasound will be passed through *B* to *C* and some will be reflected from *B* back to the transducer. Some of the ultrasound that passes through *B* will be reflected from the bottom of the cylinder, *C*, and some will continue beyond *C*. Thus, two points of reflection can be recognized, *B* and *C*. Actually, additional points can be recognized, for some of the ultrasound may re-reflect off point *A* or the transducer to points *B* and *C*. These re-echoes are known as phantom images. Phantoms are visualized as points twice as far away as the actual *B* and *C*. Similar events can occur in clinical echocardiography, and phantoms can produce a duplication of the heart, thus giving the appearance of a heart behind a heart. These must be recognized as phantoms and not considered part of the primary image.

The echocardiograph display automatically changes velocity into distance. This is accomplished by calibration; i.e., knowing speed of tissue penetration and time, depth can be calculated automatically. Since the cylinder is filled with saline, the calibration will be nearly, but not precisely, correct because the machine was calibrated for soft

Fig. 1-4. — Echoes and re-echoes. See text for the description and interpretation of the figure. The unique feature of this figure is the explanation and demonstration of re-echoes from point *A*. These frequently are called phantom images in echocardiography.

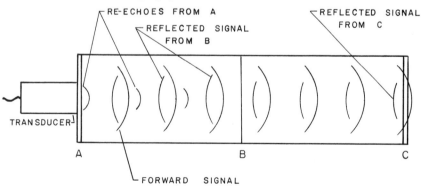

tissue, which has a velocity of 1540 m/sec, whereas saline has a velocity of 1534 m/sec. The distance between A and B, B and C and A and C thus can be read directly from the echocardiograph. The various types of displays and use of instrumentation are covered in Chapter 2.

2 / Instrumentation

BIOLOGIC SAFETY

PULSED ULTRASOUND in dosages commonly used for diagnostic work has not been reported to have produced any untoward reactions. Deleterious effects of ultrasound are due to cavitation and thermal generation. Damage is related to the duration of exposure.[210, 244] Further, ultrasound-induced damage seems to be an all-or-none phenomenon for any particular period of exposure and does not seem to be cumulative. Since ultrasound is pulsed and the pulses are very short, the average duration of exposure is very small. According to Edler *et al.*,[46] the peak sound energy intensity used in echocardiography is 40 watts/cm^2 but the average intensity is one thousand times less, or 0.04 watts/cm^2. This average intensity load is far less than that known to cause tissue damage. Ultrasound is considered so safe that it is used in obstetric scanning.

ELECTRICAL SAFETY

One possible patient hazard is electrical shock. This would occur most commonly if the patient were simultaneously exposed to two different electrical power grounds. Common second power grounds include a grounded electrocardiogram terminal, the rail of an electric bed, the metal shield of a lamp, etc. Any difference in potential between the echocardiograph ground and another instrument or appliance would pass through the patient.[229] It should be common practice to obtain power for the echo machine from the same group of power receptacles that furnish power for other services for that patient. Since an electrocardiographic monitor and the echocardiograph have low-resistance connection to the patient, the difference in potential between grounds could be of sufficient magnitude to cause cardiac fibrillation. This problem is not peculiar to echo, as it exists with any type of electrical equipment. Some echo transducers have an outer metal shell connected to a power ground. To eliminate this hazard, transducers usually are encapsulated in plastic so that no metal contacts the patient. This isolation is acceptable if the plastic does not crack or chip. Frequent inspection of the transducer will assist the echocardiographer in avoiding this hazard. Moreover, the integrity of the ground wire in the power cord and the leakage current of the instrument with and without the ground wire should be checked periodically. If the leakage current exceeds 25 microamperes, it could endanger a patient.[229] Ideally, leakage should be less than 10 microamperes. These are precautions that should be taken with any equipment used on patients.

THE OSCILLOSCOPE

An oscilloscope, frequently called a scope, permits electrical signals to be observed with respect to magnitude and phase. The signal usually progresses from left to right across the face of the scope. The information usually is displayed on the Y axis and the X axis is swept across the scope to represent time. The Z axis of the oscilloscope is the brightness of the display.

This scope display is fundamental to echocardiography, for it permits the echocardiographer to see the results of his efforts. The oscilloscope of the echograph sometimes is referred to as the echoscope.

UNDERSTANDING THE ECHOCARDIOGRAPHIC CONTROLS

GAIN. — The gain control permits an increase in the electronic signal strength of the received echoes without changing the intensity of the sound energy produced. It is similar in concept to the volume control of a phonograph. Some manufacturers use the term "attenuation" for the same function.

At least two types of gain are available on an echograph — near and total. Total gain permits a uniform increase in size of all signals (Fig. 2-1).

Ultrasound obeys the principles of sound and therefore signals diminish in intensity in proportion to the distance traveled. If total gain were the only gain available, near echoes would be large and far ones would be small. To overcome this problem, a compensation technique is used that permits gain to be increased for signals more distant from the transducer. This compensation circuit is variously called "time gain compensation" (TGC), "depth compensation" or "distance compensation." The operator can choose the starting point for increased gain and the slope at which gain will increase (Fig. 2-2).

Instruments that we have used do not permit the slope to increase rapidly enough for small infants. For an adult, the slope works well, but for the small child it does not. The slope for the infant must start and end in about 7.5 mm (Fig. 2-3). If the slope for the infant required the same 2.5 cm as shown for the adult, the entire cardiac depth of the infant would be used for the slope. We had our Smith-

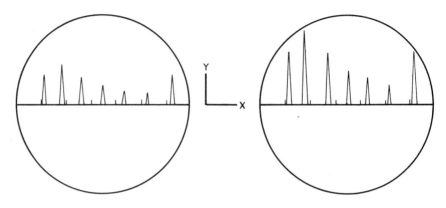

INITIAL GAIN   TOTAL GAIN INCREASED

Fig. 2-1. — The effect of an increase in signal gain (or a decrease in attenuation). The two circles depict the A-mode oscilloscopic display. Each spike represents one signal. The height of the spike in the Y axis is directly related to the amplitude of the returning echo. Distance markers are shown as uniformly spaced, equal amplitude signals with no appreciable width. The right oscilloscopic display shows the result of increasing the amplitude of each echo by an equal factor. Amplitude increment was achieved by increasing the gain of the total instrument.

Kline echograph adjusted so that a nearly vertical slope was available for the infant, but the usual slope was available also. Gain compensation is not needed for some children, but for other children and adults it is essential. No setting is universally useful and the settings of this and virtually all other controls are changed during each examination.

REJECT. — Reject is an electronic technique of eliminating low-amplitude signals. An example of rejection is shown in Figure 2-4. All signals above the selected level are retained but all smaller signals are lost. The rejection level must be variable.

Rejection eliminates echoes that arise in cavities when gain is high. The greater the gain the greater the need for reject. Less reject is required with higher-frequency transducers. At 7.5 MHz, reject rarely is used because even desirable echoes are weak.

DAMPING. — This control is not available on all echocardiographs. Electronically, it decreases the input pulse width to the transducer and thus reduces its sound energy output. This control is most useful for bringing into view detailed structures, such as endocardium.

DELAY OR START. — This control rarely is changed and sets the os-

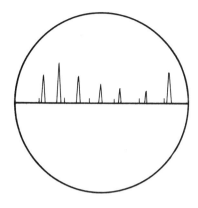 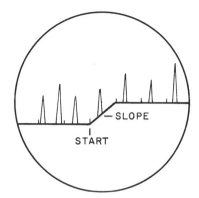

INITIAL SIGNAL   DEPTH COMPENSATION ADDED

Fig. 2-2.—The effect of depth compensation. The initial set of signals in
the left display is exactly as shown in Figure 2-1. Sound diminishes in intensity in proportion to the distance between the source and the sensor. Accordingly, more distant echoes will be represented as smaller in magnitude.
Depth compensation is used to provide amplification to these more distant
signals in order to restore them. Total instrument gain cannot be utilized for
this because the near echoes do not need similar amplification. The operator
can control the point at which the more distant echoes will be amplified by
adjusting the "start", and the rate at which the amplification will take place
by adjusting the "slope." Both functions should be nearly continuously
adjustable. The right figure shows that with depth compensation the more
distant echoes were amplified but the near signals were not. The middle echo
is on the slope, and is magnified by only 40% as much as the signals farther
to the right. When depth compensation is utilized, the near gain controls
signals to the left of the slope and the total gain is used to control the
magnitude of all signals. The depth compensation adds still more gain to
those signals on and following the slope.

cilloscope position of the "main bang," the echo representation of
the skin-transducer interface. Ideally, it should be adjustable with a
screwdriver rather than a knob, as it requires little readjustment on
instruments used exclusively for echocardiography.

SCALE EXPANSION OR DEPTH.—The total depth of field may be increased or decreased by this control. For example, the entire field
could be set to look only at the anterior wall of the right ventricle,
but this is impractical, since such a setting would exceed the resolution of the instrument. Compressing the heart into a third of the
available field is possible but is an equal error because the available
resolution is not well utilized. The most reasonable compromise is to
place the "main bang" at the top of the screen and the pericardium

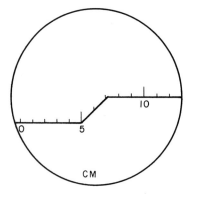 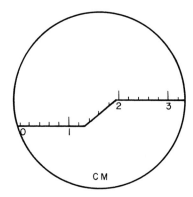

DEPTH COMPENSATION   DEPTH COMPENSATION
FOR ADULT   FOR INFANT

Fig. 2-3.—The steepness of the slope is an important consideration. The depth of an adult heart is about 10 cm, but an infant heart is only about 3 cm deep to the sternum. Thus, the slope for the infant must begin and end in 1 cm or less. The rate of rise of the slope for the adult is less critical because the heart is larger. However, some instruments cannot start and complete the slope in less than 2 cm.

Fig. 2-4.—Reject is used to eliminate low-amplitude signals. The level of rejection, shown at the dotted line, usually is variable. Any signal that has more amplitude than the rejection level will remain. All signals with amplitudes less than the rejection level will be eliminated.

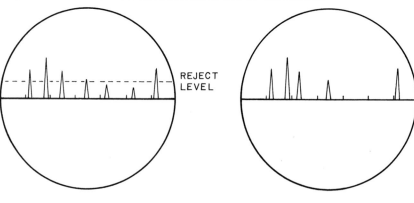

INITIAL SIGNAL   SIGNAL AFTER REJECT

1–3 cm from the bottom. This setting reasonably assumes that the entire heart will remain on the screen and a pericardial effusion will not be missed. Re-echoes, which are phantom images, are eliminated from view by this setting. These phantoms are a frequent source of error for the less experienced.

Combining the functions of delay and depth, one can place the septum or some other structure at the top of the trace and another structure, perhaps the posterior left ventricular wall, at the bottom of the trace. This technique will "lose" the right ventricle. This is the manner in which many isolated structures are photographed and appear in the literature. We find this a confusing presentation, for orientation is lost and errors can be made. An isolated mitral and tricuspid valve can appear identical but, in the context of other structures, they are identifiable. The isolation technique should be reserved for special situations.

ELECTROCARDIOGRAM GAIN AND POSITION. — An electrocardiogram is used as a timing signal. The electrocardiographic gain simply makes the signal larger on the screen. Ideally, the electrocardiogram should be positioned above the "main bang," but some instruments do not permit this, and this is a serious engineering error. If the electrocardiogram cannot be placed above the "main bang," it must be run through the echo and frequently it is lost in the myriad of structures. One constantly must move the electrocardiogram into clear areas of the trace, such as the left atrium or the right ventricle. Other systems blank out the echo around the ECG, thus sacrificing the echo, in order to show the ECG.

POLAROID PHOTOGRAPHIC CONTROLS. — These controls are used for adjustment of the echocardiograph oscilloscope, which the camera photographs. They do not affect the video output to external strip chart recorders. On the Smith-Kline unit, these are intensity, clip and sweep speed. The intensity control regulates the brightness of the entire display. On the Smith-Kline, it is properly set by adjusting the screwdriver control so that the bright line that sweeps across the scope face is decreased in intensity to the point just before it is too faint to be seen.

The "clip" control adjusts the brightness of each echo. The objective is to set this control so that very close echoes can be resolved when photographed.

Finally, the sweep speed is selected to suit the need of the examiner. For children with fast heart rates, we find that the slowest sweep speed causes too much compression of the tracing to be very valuable. Faster sweep speeds are necessary.

STORAGE OSCILLOSCOPES VS. MODERATE-PERSISTENCE OSCILLOSCOPES

The main reason for use of a storage scope is for photography. For this application, a storage tube has the advantage of holding a stationary image. Thus, one can see the image prior to photographing it and judge its acceptability. This convenience can be understood best after consideration of the photography technique of a standard oscilloscope. In the latter instance, the examiner must decide that the beats subsequent to those being viewed will be acceptable. Then a time exposure is started as the trace moves from one side of the oscilloscope to the other. Regardless of whether the child moves or the transducer sweep is not as good as the practice maneuver, the picture is already committed. Many photographs will be wasted (wastage is particularly guaranteed if children are examined).

Storage oscilloscopes are also quite useful for teaching because features of interest can be stored, examined and used as examples. It is difficult to teach with standard oscilloscopes because the images disappear quickly and unless the room is relatively dark, only one person can see the oscilloscope face at a time.

Storage scopes have serious trade-offs. Resolution usually is inferior to that of standard oscilloscopes. No gray scale is available for a standard storage tube. Since resolution is of great importance in echocardiography, the issue cannot be taken lightly. Improved storage scope resolution may be achieved at some future time. Some manufacturers provide both storage and standard oscilloscope displays in the same instrument; however, this increases cost.

An oscilloscope tube with medium to long persistence is preferable to a very short-persistence tube such as one with a P-1 phosphor. We had an "opportunity" to work with a short-persistence phosphor tube. Although it photographed well, it was virtually unusable because the total lack of an afterimage made recognition of structures nearly impossible. A commercial instrument now is available with a non-fade display, but we have had no experience with it.

HARD COPY DEVICES

Two general types of hard copy printouts are available: time exposure photographs and continuous strip recording.

Time exposure photography, usually with Polaroid pictures, has already been mentioned. This technique provides very good resolution if the focus, "f" stop and oscilloscope trace intensity are set correctly. However, performing a complete examination is difficult, if detail is important, for only several beats can be photographed. If the object is to show continuity of structures, a slow sweep can be selected. However, detail will be lost because of the slow sweep. To get a complete sweep, one often "rushes" to get it on the photo and, in so doing, may (1) miss structures and (2) introduce artifact.

Perhaps the greatest difficulty with the Polaroid technique is experienced during the photography of a pediatric echocardiogram. Younger children are *far* less likely to remain motionless during an examination than are adults. The tiniest movement of the transducer will ruin the picture. Our experience indicates that half of the pictures taken of infants and small children are wasted and many that are not wasted are of lower quality than would be desired.

We have also observed that it is difficult to train individuals to do echocardiography if the only recording technique is Polaroid. Frustrations frequently run high for examiner, child and parent.

If only a few beats are available for examination, the probability of incorrect interpretation is increased. A strip chart recording, on the other hand, permits dozens or even hundreds of consecutive beats to be examined.

Despite the drawbacks of time exposure photography, almost all of the original work with echocardiography was performed with Polaroid, and the findings from those investigations have stood the test of time.

STRIP RECORDING.—Numerous strip chart techniques are available. These can be separated into two groups:

1. Analog gate.
2. Total video displays.

The analog gate is mainly of historic interest. This technique provided the capability of selecting a single signal, usually the mitral valve, for display on a multichannel strip recording. The echocardiogram was used as a reference signal for a phonocardiogram or a pressure tracing. Obviously, display of only one of many simultaneous echoes has limited application.

Strip chart technique can permit the entire video signal and usually a reference trace to be displayed simultaneously. Since no strip chart technique is ideal, many trade-offs are present. The basic problem is that more information is available in the video signal than can be easily recorded on paper, which usually is called "hard copy." Three basic qualities contained in the video signals must be preserved: (1) accuracy of reproduction, (2) resolution and (3) gray scale.

For accuracy of reproduction, the printout must precisely reflect the video signal. The optics must not distort the image, even at the edges. Astigmatism must not be present. Linearity must be preserved. This means that 1 cm depth at the top of the printout must equal 1 cm depth at the bottom of the printout. Finally, all video information must appear on the hard copy.

Previously, resolution was defined as the ability to discriminate closely spaced echoes. Thus, the slightest focusing problem or insensitivity of the printout medium will cause small echo structures to blend into one another. Focus becomes even more critical when the echo of a newborn's heart, which is only 3 cm in depth, is expanded to cover 6 or more inches of strip chart width.

Gray scale refers to the number of shades of gray that can be distinguished between white and black. In general, the more shades of gray available the better the recording. The shade of gray is a function of the intensity of the received echo. The amplitude of an echo is a function of the degree of acoustic impedance mismatch at the interface of two structures. The brightness of each echo is roughly proportional to its amplitude. The brightness thus is reflected in the printout as a shade of gray.

Photographic film may be used as the hard copy medium. High-quality optics are available for this option and, with proper film selection, good resolution and gray scale can be accomplished. However, the end product, a continuous film strip, is difficult to use. The film is not immediately available for observation following the procedure and the examiner has no proof of his success or failure until the child has gone home, to the ward or to the bathroom. Measurements must be obtained by projecting the film onto a screen. Thus, interpretations are tedious with film strip as compared to a paper hard copy. Moreover, film processing is relatively critical, expensive and time consuming. All cardiologists involved in cineangiocardiography understand the myriad of problems encountered in processing movie film, which include improperly constituted solutions, solution temperature variations, film torn in the processor, fogging, etc. If a good film strip is obtained, reproduction onto photographic paper can result in a very-high-quality but expensive product.

A photographic process may be used that substitutes photographic paper for film. The video signal is displayed as points on the Y axis of an oscilloscope. Photographic paper is drawn at a constant rate past an optical system that focuses the row of points from the oscilloscope face onto paper. Thus, the paper drive furnishes the X axis. This system is heavily dependent on the quality of the optics and the photographic paper. The paper may be processed rapidly, so that it is available for viewing a few seconds after exposure. Alternatively, it may be rolled into a dark canister for later processing — "dark boxing." The former method provides a black on yellow-brown copy whereas the latter provides a black on white background copy. Even the rapidly developed paper requires later chemical processing. The black on white background is more pleasing to the eye than the rapidly processed record, but the immediate feedback of recognizing success or failure in recording is pleasing to the psyche. Failure to obtain a critical recording has totally disappointed us in some instances when we attempted to "dark box." In those instances, the paper had run out, torn or one of the controls had been inadvertently altered.

The photographic system is very dependent on excellent optics, and some investigators have better optical systems in their similar machines than others. The same echocardiogram recorded simultaneously on two different instruments may show vast gray scale differences.

The advantages of photographic paper recording are (1) almost immediate results if a rapid processor is used, (2) excellent linearity from top to bottom, (3) the capability of multiplexing other physiologic tracings and (4) excellent quality of photographs for publication or other presentation.

These recorders have additional disadvantages. Most are far too large to be portable. The necessity to add chemicals is a nuisance but tolerable. If used portable despite the size, the chemicals splash. The warm-up time for the rapid developer can be a serious problem if one works with children, for youngsters may not remain cooperative while the machine comes up to proper temperature. Finally, the paper processing, whether accomplished by "dark box" or rapid development, requires considerable technician time.

Another class of recorder permits paper or film to be drawn over a fiberoptic column that is attached to the oscilloscope face. The Honeywell 1856 is such an instrument. The fiberoptic column is composed of many thousands of fibers that conduct light. The principal advantage of this system is the avoidance of a lens, which is made possible because the light images are carried directly from the oscilloscope face to the paper by the fibers. If the oscilloscope is in focus, the image on the paper will be in focus. The paper will also receive all of the gray scale that the oscilloscope is capable of rendering and thus the gray scale of the paper becomes an important determinant. The resolution of this system should be superior, and we have found this to be true. Most commonly, ultraviolet paper is the hard copy medium for this recorder, although photographic film or photographic paper could be used. Ultraviolet paper develops in ultraviolet light almost instantly and does not require further processing. Some ultraviolet paper is available that can also be chemically processed to produce a white on black image. If the ultraviolet paper is left in ambient light for long periods, the trace tends to fade. This can be speeded immeasurably by xeroxing traces. Even in the absence of light, the trace degrades after long periods, but tracings made with ultraviolet paper 10 years ago still are readable. The Honeywell recorder is relatively small, and we use it almost exclusively as a portable instrument. Since it is relatively light in weight, we also take it with us to field clinics and other hospitals in the city.

Ultraviolet paper has several other disadvantages. The blue on brown tracing is not as aesthetically pleasing as black on white. Fading in ambient light and with time is a relative problem. Ultraviolet paper costs no less than conventional photographic paper. Photographing ultraviolet hard copy is more difficult than photographing black on white or white on black. However, almost all echocardiograms in this book were obtained with a Honeywell recorder and ultraviolet paper. The expense of the fiberoptic recorder is greater than the expense of most photographic recorders. Finally, one must purchase expensive multiplexers if additional traces other than the electrocardiogram are to be presented simultaneously on the echocardiogram. In most instances, adding channels to the conventional photographic paper machine is less expensive.

Ultraviolet paper has one additional benefit that does not relate to the quality of the tracing. A thin base paper is available, which, when folded, decreases storage space requirements considerably as compared to conventional photographic paper.

Another recording instrument, somewhat similar in concept to the Honeywell recorder, has been marketed. This is a thermal recorder that lacks the resolution of the Honeywell instrument. Some units had the disadvantage of nonlinearity. Resolution is relatively limited. This instrument apparently is being phased out and will not be discussed in detail.

WAYS OF DISPLAYING THE ECHOCARDIOGRAM

It will be recalled from Chapter 1 that the amplitude of a returning echo is a function of the impedance mismatch of the interface that created the reflection. In the A-mode, the amplitude of the echo is transformed into a spike, and the height of the spike is a function of the amplitude. A-mode is useful for stationary echoes, but recording of moving echoes is technically difficult in this mode. To overcome this, the amplitude of a spike can be converted into a point

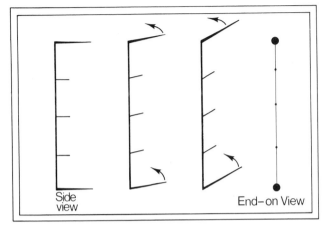

A ⟶ B – MODE

Fig. 2-5. – Conceptualization of conversion of A-mode to B-mode (see text for details).

of light. The brightness of the point of light is made roughly proportional to the amplitude of the echo. Figure 2-5 shows diagrammatically that the A-mode can be mentally converted to the B-mode by rotating the display 90° with respect to the viewer. This is best thought of as looking at the A-mode spikes "on end." The electronic methodology used to obtain B-mode from A-mode is, of course, quite different. Then, if the B-mode is recurrently swept across the oscilloscope, changes in structure depth with respect to time can be observed. This technique is the M-mode.

ECHO MODES. – Figure 2-6 diagrammatically summarizes the echo display concept. Since cardiac anatomy has not been discussed, a more familiar sonar concept will be used.

In panel *A*, a ship is moving from the right side of the picture to the left. Its transducer (xdcr) is pulsing echoes through a homogeneous medium, sea water, which has a sound transmission of approximately 1535 m/sec. Four miles below is an interface perpendicular to the echo beam, the ocean floor. Echoes are seen reflecting off the ocean floor and returning to the transducer.

The oscilloscope displays are shown below in the A, B and M-modes. Entering the scene will be a treasure chest and later a fish undulating at different depths as he swims along.

In vertical panel *A*, we note that 1 centimeter equals 1 mile. On the A-mode, the first spike, TB, represents transducer bang. The next spike, OF, represents the ocean floor. The velocity of sound through

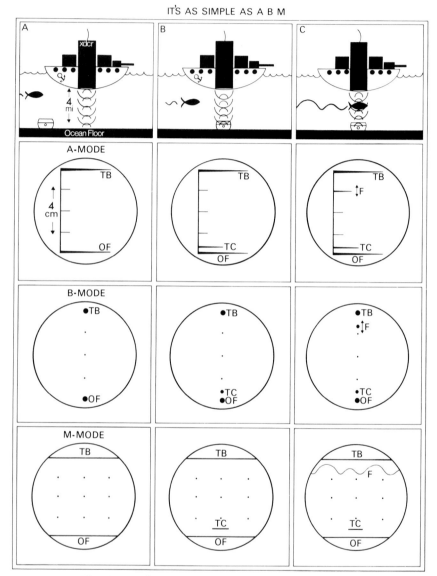

Fig. 2-6. — The sonar principle (see text for details).

the sea water and the time from transducer output of sound to reception of returning echoes are used to calibrate the oscilloscope display (1 cm = 1 mile). Thus, the ocean floor is found to be 4 miles deep.

The B-mode shows these spikes as stationary large dots separated by 4 cm, which equals 4 miles. The calibration lines from the A-mode now are seen as calibration dots.

The M-mode display shows the two large dots from the B-mode swept across the scope. Since there is no depth change, they are represented as two lines. The calibration dots are recorded every ½ second.

In panel B, the ship has moved farther to the left and now passes over the treasure chest (TC). Some sound is reflected from the surface of the chest, and a new spike, TC, is seen on the A-mode display. Some sound passes through the chest. Therefore, the OF spike still is present. The fish is closer but not yet encountered by the sonar beam. The previous parameters and the treasure chest now are displayed in the B-mode.

The advantage of the M-mode now is apparent. To see the chest on A or B we must photograph or store the image at that encounter point in time. On the M-mode, we record the appearance of the treasure chest as the transducer passes over it. A picture in the A-mode or B-mode would include TC only if that picture were timed to coincide with the passage of the ship over the chest.

In panel C, we repeat the ship's passage over the treasure chest and also observe that the undulating fish has found his way into the echo beam. Sound passes through and reflects from the fish, the treasure chest and the ocean floor.

The A-mode display shows a moving spike, F, which represents the fish's up-and-down motion. The TC spike then is seen, a bit more prominently than the spike of the soft tissue fish. The heavy ocean floor spike is then recorded. If this were photographed, the concept of the moving fish spike would be lost. Thus, photographing A-mode is useful for stationary structures.

The B-mode shows the heavy TB dot, a moving fish dot, a TC dot and a heavy OF dot, 4 miles deep. Again, if photographed, this would not show motion. If we were examining a cavity that contained fairly stationary objects, such as a pregnant uterus or an abdominal cavity, and if multiple planes of examination were stored on an oscilloscope face and then photographed, this composite would give a good representation of depth, location and size of such structures as kidneys, liver, tumors, aorta, cysts, placentae or fetuses. This is the application in B-mode scanning.

If B-mode is swept across an oscilloscope, the undulating motion of the fish is observed, thus M (motion)-mode. The velocity and depth of his movements can be plotted. The TC and OF are seen as before. OF is a constant line and the TC is observed in its length and depth as the transducer is smoothly swept across it. M-mode is used in cardiac study because it can capture moving structures, such as valves, heart walls or vessels.

TRANSPORTATION FOR THE ECHOGRAPH

At first glance, a portable cart seems to be a minor issue, but it is not. Instrumentation portability is extremely important. The echocardiograph must be able to go where the action is—the operating, recovery or emergency room, the catheterization laboratory or the ward. The objective of the cart is to get the echograph to the patient safely, conveniently and rapidly. Once the equipment has arrived, the cart should permit the instrument to be used with as much facility as possible.

We found no suitable commercially available cart and were forced to build one. We desired a cart with the following features:

1. It should be no longer than necessary and narrow enough to fit between beds.

2. It should have considerable enclosed storage space.

3. Instruments should be protected against slippage.

4. It should have large ball bearing wheels so that wheels will not become wedged when entering or leaving elevators.

5. It should be easily steered by even the smallest technician.

Our cart, with echograph and recorder, is shown in Figure 2-7, A.

No obvious advantage is afforded by a cart that tilts the instrument upward. Since the oscilloscope is elevated by this tilt, one must find a high stool or stand while doing the test. We prefer to have the oscilloscope and instrument flat and at eye level when sitting in a standard chair. If one uses a Honeywell 1856, the echograph must sit above the echo recorder because the reverse arrangement will cause the paper to fall over the controls of the echoscope. Cart height should take this into account.

If the user plans to transport the echograph to clinics outside the hospital, a folding portable cart is necessary because available carts are too large to fit into an automobile. We had the experience of having a loaner cart collapse and cause the echocardiograph to crash to the floor. Fortunately, it was not damaged. Since that episode, we

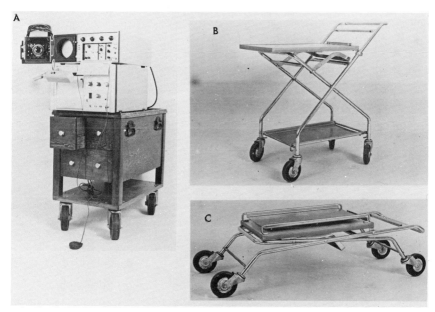

Fig. 2-7.—A shows a Smith-Kline Echoline 20A placed on top of a Honeywell 1856. Both instruments are mounted on a mobile cart. B and C show a collapsible cart that we use for portable work outside our base hospital. Its principal asset is that it will fit into an automobile trunk.

obtained a very sturdy collapsible portable cart with large wheels (Fig. 2-7, B and C). This selection permitted the echograph, recorder and collapsed cart to fit into the trunk of a compact car. It could be used as a permanent cart, but it has no storage space or guard rails to prevent the instrument from slipping.

If portability is an important issue, instrument size becomes a major consideration. From an electronics state-of-the-art consideration, all echocardiographs manufactured at this time are physically too large. Ideally, the instrument should be no larger than an electrocardiographic monitor or a small oscilloscope. Integrated circuitry could provide this benefit, but few size changes have been made since the instruments were introduced to the medical market a number of years ago.

The portable electronic instrument must be ruggedly designed. Constant transportation on carts, airplanes or in automobile trunks probably will take its toll. Fortunately, we have experienced only one serious instrument breakdown outside the hospital in more than 70 trips, some of which were for hundreds of miles. However, our repair department has found numerous parts that have become "loose." Periodic preventive maintenance is extremely important if the instrument is to remain functional.

IRRITATING FEATURES OF SOME INSTRUMENTS: CAVEAT EMPTOR!

1. An electrocardiogram that cannot be placed above the "main bang."

2. A focus control placed on the back of the instrument so as to require adjustment with a mirror in a dark room.

3. A frequency switch on the back of the instrument.

4. No damping control.

5. An interrupt when viewing M-mode. Some instruments have a significant delay period between each sweep. One cannot continuously look at the trace, for it goes blank after every sweep for a few seconds. This is very frustrating with any patient, but particularly so with a squirmy infant.

6. An instrument meant to be observed only in the A-mode. The only M-mode display occurs during time exposure photography.

7. An instrument that requires refocusing when switching from A-mode to M-mode. This is particularly a problem when combined with problem 2.

8. An instrument that has a very short-persistence phosphor tube, such as a P-1. This makes echocardiography virtually impossible.

9. An instrument that will not permit use of high-frequency transducers.

10. An instrument with excessive knobs.

11. A sweep that proceeds from bottom to top of the oscilloscope rather than from left to right. In some instruments this is quickly remedied by rotating the oscilloscope tube 90°.

3 / The Normal Echocardiogram

THE ECHOCARDIOGRAPHIC EXAMINATION concentrates on planes of study that may, at first, seem awkward or slightly unfamiliar to physicians or technicians. These planes are dictated by the areas of the precordium that are free of overlying lung and bone, for the ultrasonic beam is virtually totally reflected by the lung and considerably attenuated by bone. We are limited to a transducer location that is a few centimeters wide and extends from the second to the fourth interspace. Initially, it may appear that viewing the heart through such a relatively small window would not permit adequate examination. However, consider watching a baseball game through a knothole in a fence. If the fence is far from the playing field, the entire game can be seen. The observer may not see a few far left or far right bleacher seats or structures very close to the knothole, but an accurate idea of the baseball game can be obtained.

Figure 5-2 shows the fulcrum effect of the transducer on beam passage. Envision a long-bladed knife with a short handle. A slight angulation of the handle will create a large sweep of the tip of the blade. The same applies to the echocardiographic beam. Despite the limited window, most of the heart can be visualized by sweeping the beam. Structures that are recorded most easily are those farthest from the fulcrum, such as the left ventricle, the left atrium and the ascending aorta. Indeed, the entire length of these structures usually can be recorded by a slight transducer angulation. Closer structures, such as the anterior right ventricular wall and cavity, on the other hand, are more difficult to visualize because only a small portion of these structures are intersected by the echo beam.

Cardiac chambers, septae, walls and great vessels have been identified by pressure or hand injection of indocyanine green dye, saline or blood at the time of cardiac catheterization.[92] It is postulated that injection of these solutions produces a shower of microbubbles. The microbubbles cause multiple echoes in the chamber under study. These bubbles pass with the flow of blood, and subsequent chambers or vessels can be visualized also. However, the microbubbles do not seem to pass through the lung. Once cardiac structures were so identified, they could be characterized by their motions, size, position and depth. It no longer is necessary to inject solutions because usually positioned structures can be recognized by their various

characteristics. However, patients with marked anatomic derangement still may require injection of solution for absolute identification
of structures.

Although cardiac structures can be recognized, the availability of
normal quantitative values for these structures is limited for the pediatric patient. Some groups have studied the neonate, and their
data for structural thickness, dimension and mobility will be included.[153, 97, 212] However, no large series of data was available for subjects beyond the neonatal period. To fill this void, we performed a
study of the normal child. Our study group consisted of 100 normal
healthy children who had echocardiograms while attending a well-
child clinic. All measurements were confirmed by three independent
observers. Feigenbaum and Konecke[56] kindly permitted us to pool
their normal data with ours. They had investigated 103 normal children at Indiana University. Thus, our combined series represents
about 200 for most values. A few of the variables were not measured
in the Indiana group. In these instances, the series is only half as
large, containing only the Arizona data. We compared our data to
Indiana's for each structure and for each 0.2 m² increment in body
surface area. The two sets of data are statistically similar except for
the smallest left atrial measurements. The Arizona measurements of
the left atrium are consistently smaller than the Indiana measurements in the body surface area groups between 0.3 and 0.8 m². The
reason for this discrepancy is that the Indiana left atrial measurements
included the width of the posterior aortic wall. The left atrial measurements are the same.above 0.8 m².

We arranged the compiled data by comparing each measured parameter to body surface area. Linear, logarithmic and root correla-
tions were evaluated. We selected the highest correlation coefficient
relationship for display in this chapter. Some biologic data are not
normally distributed in the general population. As our data are no
exception to this principle, we selected the fifth, fiftieth and ninety-
fifth percentiles for presentation. Standard deviations above and below the mean would have little value.

GENERAL CONCEPT OF THE ECHOCARDIOGRAM

The diagrammatic echo part of Figure 3-1 was conceived by Feigenbaum to explain longitudinal echocardiographic anatomy in the
planes most commonly used in the echocardiographic examination.
Cardiac sections in the planes viewed are shown below the diagram
and labeled structures of the composite section are at the right.

The echocardiogram is interpreted as starting at the top with the "main bang," which is a thick line representing the skin-transducer interface. Each structure is recorded with respect to its depth from the transducer. The echocardiogram permits an orderly sequence for viewing the heart. Each anatomic structure has its own characteristic location and movement and each plane of examination has its own significance.

The single crystal echocardiogram usually is interpreted as a sum of parts rather than as a whole. Individual structures are evaluated with respect to a reference structure and a composite impression is formed. Limitations are present because anatomic structural depths can necessitate different instrument settings for emphasis of particular cardiac areas. It is thus unusual to have a perfect single picture for all structures during every examination, but the best possible complete composite echocardiogram should be sought during every examination. What is left out one day can haunt the next.

Echocardiograms are qualitative and quantitative. Quantitation will be stressed, for it is essential and too frequently is forgotten in the maze of qualitative data. Measurement often is accomplished with calipers. We also use a variable-length calibrated spring ruler, which provides excellent accuracy and speeds measurement.

Calibration markers are provided by the echograph as intermittent dots or lines. Unfortunately, calibration dots or lines have width. Therefore, one always must measure the calibration marker from the top of one to the top of the other, or from bottom to bottom, but never from the top of one marker to the bottom of another. If a calibrated spring ruler is used, match the spring markers to the calibration markers for the full width of the tracing to ensure maximal accuracy.

In most commercial echographs, the usual standard of calibration is 1 centimeter in the Y axis. The distance in the X axis between calibration markers is a unit of time, usually 0.5 seconds in echocardiography. This may vary from machine to machine. If studies require accurate timing, check the timing marker's accuracy on the echograph against a known timing device.

END SYSTOLE AND END DIASTOLE

Standardization of measurement of the echocardiogram is essential if users are to communicate with one another. Authors of publications are not always clear as to when or where their measurements were made. Most authors concentrate on end systolic or end diastolic measurements, but when do these events actually occur in the child? Some standardization needs to be initiated.

We have adopted the following convention for the child. We de-

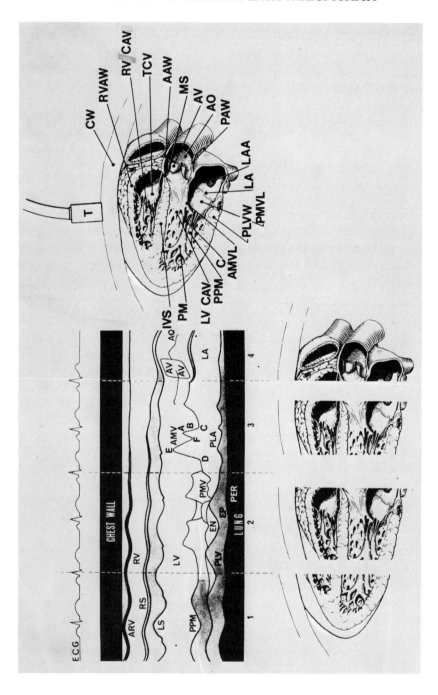

Fig. 3-1. – Echocardiographic and anatomic representations, longitudinal cardiac view. A diagram of echocardiographic patterns found in different areas of the heart is in the upper left panel. Above is an electrocardiogram for timing purposes. A composite drawing of the heart in the same plane is to the right. Beneath the echocardiographic diagram are sections of the composite that correspond to the numbered areas: *Area 1* – apex-papillary muscle plane; *Area 2* – chordae, posterior mitral leaflet plane; *Area 3* – anterior mitral leaflet plane; *Area 4* – aortic valve-left atrial plane. See text for details. Abbreviations: *ECG* = electrocardiogram; *ARV, RVAW* = anterior right ventricular wall; *RV CAV, RV* = right ventricle cavity; *TCV* = tricuspid valve; *RS* = right septal surface; *IVS* = interventricular septum; *LS* = left septal surface; *LV, LV CAV* = left ventricular cavity; *PM* = anterior papillary muscle; *PPM* = posterior papillary muscle; *C* = chordae; *AMV, AMVL* = anterior mitral valve leaflet; *PMV* = posterior mitral valve leaflet; *PLVW, PLV* = posterior left ventricular wall; *EN* = endocardium; *EP* = epicardium; *PER* = pericardium; *A, B, C, D, E, F* = points and slopes of anterior mitral valve leaflet motion; *LA* = left atrium; *LAA* = left atrial appendage; *MS* = membranous septum; *AAW* = anterior aortic wall; *AV* = aortic valve; *AO* = aorta; *PAW* = posterior aortic wall, *CW* = chest wall. (*Upper left panel* modified from Feigenbaum.[56])

fine end diastole as the first rapid motion of the electrocardiographic QRS complex. We recognize that cardiac muscle does not contract as soon as the first part of the QRS is inscribed. Others have defined end diastole and end systole with respect to the echocardiographic mitral valve opening and closing movements.[195] This has merit for left ventricular events, but tricuspid closure usually is slightly later than mitral.

Some individuals who deal with adult patients incorporate the concept of electromechanical lag by performing their measurement a period of time after the QRS complex; for example, 40 milliseconds. However, the QRS complex is shorter in duration in the child than in the adult. If we were to delay our measurement by 40 milliseconds in all children, a different set of circumstances would be introduced in children of different ages. It is for these reasons that we make end diastolic measurements in a uniform manner, at the beginning of the QRS.

CHEST WALL

The "main bang," which represents the skin-transducer interface, is at the top of the echocardiogram. It usually is recorded as a thick line (Fig. 3-2). This is not a structure but an interface. The first structure encountered by the penetrating beam is the anterior chest wall. Its thickness varies from individual to individual. It usually is represented as a homogeneous stationary structure. Details of specific layers of the chest wall are not germane to the cardiac examination.

ANTERIOR PERICARDIUM

The next structure encountered by the echo beam is the anterior pericardium. This structure usually does not move and adheres to the right ventricular wall. It is observed infrequently in the normal and more often in a patient with a pericardial effusion.

In 10% of our normal series, the pericardium was separated from the right ventricular anterior wall, the left ventricular posterior wall or both. These separations occur during systole and may be due to the presence of normal pericardial fluid, particularly if they occur posteriorly.

RIGHT VENTRICULAR ANTERIOR WALL

The right ventricular anterior wall lies below the anterior pericardium. It contracts after the electrocardiographic QRS complex. It is measured at end diastole in the plane that simultaneously shows the posterior leaflet of the mitral valve (Fig. 3-2). This may seem to be a rather unusual constraint for right ventricular measurement, but it does represent a degree of logic. The objective is to measure the right ventricle in a repeatable area. The posterior mitral valve leaflet is a small structure and sighting it markedly limits the area of the right ventricle subtended by the echo beam, particularly if the transducer is nearly perpendicular and located about midway over the precordium. Therefore, approximately the same portion of the right ventricle will be evaluated each time.

Visualization of the right ventricular anterior wall by echocardiography may be difficult. Therefore, a comment on avoiding errors is in order. The right ventricle must be specifically sought during evaluation. The technique for this is described in detail in Chapter 5. Briefly, the near gain control must be adjusted so that the specific contractions and endocardial surface of the right ventricle are observed. Switching to the highest-frequency transducer that will permit penetration often elucidates such anterior structures as the right ventricular anterior wall, cavity and septum. These may be otherwise unresolvable. However, use of the high-frequency transducer may sacrifice clear visualization of posterior structures. This is permissible as long as the measurement plane is continuously demonstrated to be proper. A beautiful posterior mitral valve leaflet is not required, but a recognizable one is necessary in order to be certain that the plane of right ventricular anterior wall measurement is correct. Figure 3-3, A demonstrates poor visualization of the right ventricular anterior wall and Figure 3-3, B shows the right ventricular anterior wall resolved with a higher-frequency transducer. Note that this transducer change partially sacrificed the quality but not the recognition of left ventricular structures and the mitral valve. Similar transducer techniques and principles apply to the right ventricular cavity.

At present, diastolic right ventricular wall thickness is the only standardized anterior right ventricular wall measurement. Patients with various lesions and contractile status have varying degrees of systolic fiber shortening, but this has not been well studied by echocardiography, especially in the right ventricle. Exercise, digitalis and other inotropic drugs might be expected to increase contractility of the right ventricular anterior wall.

It is important to recognize that the normal right ventricle frequently separates from the chest wall during systole. If resolution is poor, the systolic thickness may appear to be from endocardium to chest wall, but this thickness may include the systolic separation.

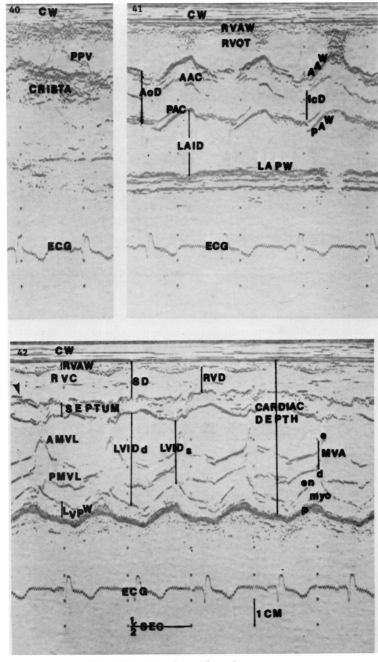

Fig. 3-2. — See legend on facing page.

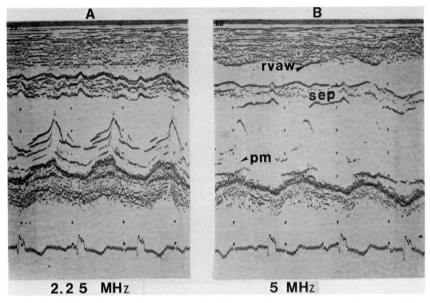

Fig. 3-3.—The echocardiogram at the left shows poor resolution of the right ventricular anterior wall. The echocardiogram at the right is from the same patient with a higher-frequency transducer being employed (5 MHz vs. 2.25 MHz). Note loss of echo penetration but cleaner anterior resolution. The echo is in the plane of the posterior mitral valve leaflet.

Fig. 3-2.—Composite echocardiogram. The upper left panel is a view of the pulmonary valve. The upper right panel is an echocardiogram taken in the plane of the aortic leaflets, which visualizes the right ventricular outflow tract, the aorta with its valve and the left atrial cavity. The lines shown (aortic dimension, intercusp distance and left atrial internal dimension) represent the phase of the cardiac cycle and location where these measurements are made. The bottom panel is an echocardiogram in the plane of the posterior mitral valve leaflet. The arrow points to part of the tricuspid apparatus, which is frequently confused with the right septal surface. Again, the lines shown represent various measurements and their timing. These include right ventricular anterior wall, right ventricular dimension, septal depth, cardiac depth, septal thickness, left ventricular posterior wall, left ventricular internal dimension during systole and diastole and the D–E anterior mitral valve amplitude. Note that the calibration markers are 1 cm apart in the Y axis and ½ second apart in the X axis. Abbreviations: Same as in Figure 3-1 plus PPV = posterior pulmonary valve; $RVOT$ = right ventricular outflow tract; AOD = aortic dimension; AAC = anterior aortic cusp; PAC = posterior aortic cusp; IcD = intercusp distance; $LAPW$ = left atrial posterior wall; RVC = right ventricular cavity; RVD = right ventricular dimension; $LVID_d$ = left ventricular internal dimension in diastole; $LVID_s$ = left ventricular internal dimension in systole; myo = myocardium.

TABLE 3-1.—RIGHT VENTRICULAR ANTERIOR WALL THICKNESS
(DIASTOLIC) (IN CM)
Neonates

	HAGAN	SOLINGER				
	n = 200	n = 21	n = 28	n = 25	n = 22	n = 23
Weight	m = 7.6 lb	2.27 kg	2.73 kg	3.18 kg	3.64 kg	4.09 kg
Range	0.20–0.47	0.11–0.29	0.13–0.31	0.16–0.34	0.18–0.36	0.20–0.38
Mean	0.30 ± 0.01	0.20	0.22	0.25	0.27	0.29

Right ventricular wall thickness usually is constant and measures approximately 3 mm after the neonatal period. Normal measurements are presented in Table 3-1 and Figure 3-4.

RIGHT VENTRICULAR CAVITY

Deep to the anterior right ventricular wall is the right ventricular cavity (Figs. 3-1 and 3-2). When the transducer is angled through the next examining planes, 2 and 3, the right ventricular body is record-

Fig. 3-4.—Right ventricular anterior wall thickness measurement (root function). The fifth, fiftieth and ninety-fifty percentiles of the normal group described in the text are shown. The abscissa is body surface area expressed in meters squared. The ordinate is expressed in centimeters. The standard error of the estimate, p and r values are shown in the lower right portion of the graph. Note that there is very little change in thickness with age.

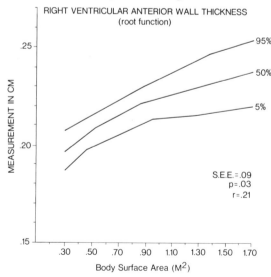

RIGHT VENTRICULAR ANTERIOR WALL THICKNESS
(root function)

S.E.E.=.09
p=.03
r=.21

TABLE 3-2.—RIGHT VENTRICULAR CAVITY (DIASTOLIC) (IN CM)

(A) Neonates and Infants

	HAGAN	MEYER		SOLINGER				FEIGENBAUM
Weight	n = 200 m = 7.6 lb	n = 50 m = 3.2 kg	n = 21 2.27 kg	n = 28 2.73 kg	n = 25 3.18 kg	n = 22 3.64 kg	n = 23 4.09 kg	n = 26 0–25 lb m = 17 lb
Range	0.61–1.50	1.0–1.7	1.04–1.46	1.10–1.52	1.16–1.58	1.23–1.65	1.29–1.71	0.3–1.5
Mean	1.14 ± 0.04	1.3	1.25	1.31	1.37	1.44	1.50	0.9

(B) Older Children

	FEIGENBAUM				
Weight	n = 26 25–50 lb m = 39 lb	n = 20 50–75 lb m = 62 lb	n = 15 75–100 lb m = 89 lb	n = 11 100–125 lb m = 113 lb	n = 5 125–200 lb m = 165 lb
Range	0.4–1.5	0.7–1.8	0.7–1.6	0.8–1.7	1.2–1.7
Mean	1.0	1.1	1.2	1.3	1.3

ed. If the beam is directed cephalad, through part of plane 3 and through plane 4, a part of the right ventricular outflow tract is transected.

In the normal subject, right ventricular volume is affected by respiration. Inspiration increases negative intrathoracic pressure and thus causes more blood to flow into the right ventricle. Expiration has the opposite effect. Rhythmic alteration in right ventricular dimension probably is due to this respiratory factor. The echocardiogram reflects this as a change in right ventricular dimension with respiration. The effect varies from hardly noticeable in normals to moderate in dyspneic babies or patients with cystic fibrosis.

The echo beam (in plane 2, Fig. 3-1) may traverse various parts of the body of the right ventricle. Much of the right ventricular body is substernal, and the area evaluated by echocardiography usually is left parasternal and more toward the right ventricular apex and outflow tract.

Normal (diastolic) measurements of the right ventricular cavity are given in Table 3-2 and Figure 3-5. This probably is the least consistent dimension encountered in echocardiography because of respiratory variation and the unusual geometry of the chamber.

Fig. 3-5.—Right ventricular cavity measurement (root function). The axes and abbreviations are the same as for Figure 3-4.

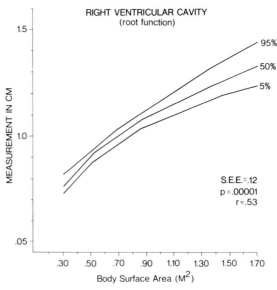

RIGHT VENTRICULAR CAVITY
(root function)

95%

50%

5%

S.E.E.=.12
p =.00001
r =.53

MEASUREMENT IN CM

Body Surface Area (M^2)

INTERVENTRICULAR SEPTUM

The interventricular septum is the next structure encountered by the penetrating beam (Figs. 3-1 and 3-2). It is continuous with and tethered to the anterior aortic wall. Additionally, it is tethered to the cardiac apex. The septum has two surfaces — right ventricular and left ventricular.

The upper portion of the septum is attached to the aorta. Multi-crystal echocardiography (see Chapter 7) shows that this portion of the septum moves with the aorta. The muscular portion of the septum below the aorta and in the plane of the posterior mitral valve leaflet has a different motion. In systole, this portion contracts with the left ventricular posterior wall as part of circumferential fiber shortening. Farther down the septal surface and toward the cardiac apex, the septum also contracts posteriorly with systole. In the child, the papillary muscles fill in this apical area of the left ventricle, further complicating examination of the septum and the posterior wall.

Septal motion and measurement must be evaluated in a consistent plane. Simultaneous sighting of the posterior mitral valve leaflet with the transducer near the perpendicular satisfies this requirement because the leaflet is small and deep to the septum (Fig. 3-1). Thus, the site of septal measurement is limited and repeatable. Care must be taken to adequately define the right ventricular septal surface for measurement purposes. Extraneous echoes as the result of insufficient rejection and echoes of the septal leaflet of the tricuspid valve or of the chordae may be confused with the right septal surface. The latter is one of the most common sources of echocardiographic interpretive error (beat 1 in Fig. 3-2).

The septum contracts after the electrocardiographic QRS complex and just before left ventricular posterior wall contraction. The contractions of the septum and the posterior wall are due to circumferential fiber shortening and act to constrict the left ventricular cavity. This causes expulsion of blood during systole. Since the mid and apical septum contracts toward the left ventricular posterior wall during systole, it must contract away from the right ventricular anterior wall.

The entire left ventricle moves anteriorly in late systole and posteriorly at the beginning of ventricular relaxation. A notch is found on the posterior septal surface toward the end of systole (Fig. 3-2). McDonald[150, 151] indicated that this notch is the result of summation of movement of the left ventricular posterior wall, the rotation of the

TABLE 3-3.—SEPTAL THICKNESS (DIASTOLIC) (IN CM)

(A) Neonates and Infants

	HAGAN	SOLINGER					FEIGENBAUM
Weight	n = 200 m = 7.6 lb	n = 21 2.27 kg	n = 28 2.73 kg	n = 25 3.18 kg	n = 22 3.64 kg	n = 23 4.09 kg	n = 26 0–25 lb m = 17 lb
Range	0.18–0.40	0.21–0.33	0.24–0.36	0.26–0.38	0.29–0.41	0.31–0.43	0.4–0.6
Mean	0.27 ± 0.004	0.27	0.30	0.32	0.35	0.37	0.5

(B) Older Children

	FEIGENBAUM				
Weight	n = 26 25–50 lb m = 39 lb	n = 20 50–75 lb m = 62 lb	n = 15 75–100 lb m = 89 lb	n = 11 100–125 lb m = 113 lb	n = 5 125–200 lb m = 165 lb
Range	0.5–0.7	0.6–0.7	0.7–0.8	0.7–0.8	0.7–0.8
Mean	0.6	0.7	0.7	0.7	0.8

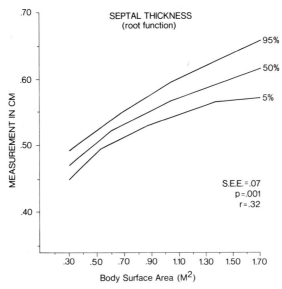

Fig. 3-6.—Septal thickness measurement (root function). The axes and abbreviations are the same as for Figure 3-4. See text for details.

left ventricle as a whole and the individual motion of the septum.

Septal diastolic measurement ordinarily equals left ventricular posterior wall measurement. Normal data for the septum are given in Table 3-3 and Figure 3-6.

AORTA

As the transducer beam is passed cephalad, the anterior aortic wall is noted to be continuous with the interventricular septum (Figs. 3-1, 3-2 and 5-7). The aortic wall is thinner than the septum and moves parallel to the posterior aortic wall. The motion is anterior in systole and posterior in diastole. It is interesting to note that there is little, if any, systolic expansion of the aortic dimension even though the flow is pulsatile. This confirms Womersley's hypothesis that there is little radial enlargement of the aortic root during systole and little contraction during diastole.[243]

Aortic root measurements are made at the beginning of the QRS complex in the section of the aorta that permits simultaneous visualization of the aortic anterior and posterior walls and the aortic valve (Fig. 3-2). Our convention is to measure the aorta from outside wall

TABLE 3-4.—Aortic Root Diameter (Diastolic) (in cm)

(A) Neonates and Infants

	Hagan	Meyer			Solinger			Feigenbaum
Weight	n = 200 m = 7.6 lb	n = 50 m = 3.2 kg	n = 21 2.27 kg	n = 28 2.73 kg	n = 25 3.18 kg	n = 22 3.64 kg	n = 23 4.09 kg	n = 26 0–25 lb m = 17 lb
Range	0.81–1.2	0.7–1.2	0.93–1.13	0.97–1.17	1.02–1.22	1.07–1.27	1.11–1.31	0.7–1.7
Mean	1.0 ± .006	1.0	1.03	1.07	1.12	1.17	1.21	1.3

(B) Older Children

Feigenbaum

Weight	n = 26 25–50 lb m = 39 lb	n = 20 50–75 lb m = 62 lb	n = 15 75–100 lb m = 89 lb	n = 11 100–125 lb m = 113 lb	n = 5 125–200 lb m = 165 lb
Range	1.3–2.2	1.7–2.3	1.9–2.7	1.7–2.7	2.2–2.8
Mean	1.7	2.0	2.2	2.3	2.4

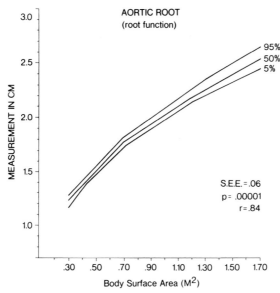

Fig. 3-7. — Aortic root measurement (root function). The axes and abbreviations are the same as for Figure 3-4.

to outside wall at end diastole. Normal values are given in Table 3-4 and Figure 3-7.

AORTIC VALVE

The echocardiographic representation of the aortic valve is located within the two aortic walls at the aortic annulus, just beyond the point where the septum joins the anterior aortic wall. Aortic valve cusps are named for the coronary arteries from which they originate and not by their location. There is controversy about which aortic cusp is viewed by echocardiography. Gramiak and Shah[90] state that the right coronary (anterior) and the noncoronary (posterior) cusps are viewed. Feigenbaum[56] is less certain and refers to them only as anterior and posterior. In view of the present lack of certainty concerning these echo representations, we subscribe to the latter terminology. Usually, the aortic valves open abruptly, stay open during systole as parallel lines and close abruptly. During diastole, they appear fused as a single line of closure.

Fine vibrations of the aortic cusps occur in systole, and presumably this is due to rapid blood flow across them. Instrumentation resolution and repetition rate also contribute to the appearance of "vibration."

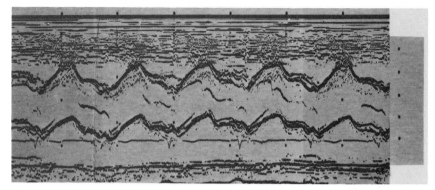

Fig. 3-8.—Echocardiogram in plane of aortic leaflets (normal patient). This echocardiogram demonstrates that the aortic diastolic closure line can be normocentric or eccentric in the same normal individual. Note the variable position of the diastolic closure line. This phenomenon is induced by transducer positioning. Calibration markers are at the right.

During systole, a third line frequently is observed bisecting the open cusps. We do not know what this line represents. That the third line is the third cusp seems unlikely, as the leaflet should be away from the center of the aorta during systole. Is it a phantom image?

The aortic valve is closed during diastole and is represented as a single line. In the normal, this line is central in the aorta or can be

TABLE 3-5.—AORTIC CUSP SEPARATION (SYSTOLIC) (IN CM)
(A) Neonates and Infants

	SOLINGER					FEIGENBAUM
Weight	n = 21 2.27 kg	n = 28 2.73 kg	n = 25 3.18 kg	n = 22 3.64 kg	n = 23 4.09 kg	n = 26 0–25 lb m = 17 lb
Range	0.40–0.54	0.43–0.57	0.45–0.59	0.48–0.62	0.51–0.65	0.5–1.2
Mean	0.47	0.50	0.52	0.55	0.58	0.9

(B) Older Children

	FEIGENBAUM				
Weight	n = 26 25–50 lb m = 39 lb	n = 20 50–75 lb m = 62 lb	n = 15 75–100 lb m = 89 lb	n = 11 100–125 lb m = 113 lb	n = 5 125–200 lb m = 165 lb
Range	0.9–1.6	1.2–1.7	1.3–1.9	1.4–2.0	1.6–2.0
Mean	1.2	1.4	1.6	1.7	1.8

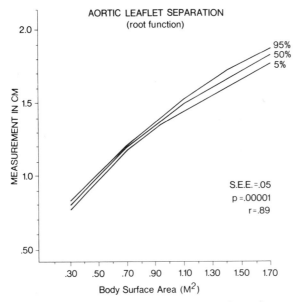

Fig. 3-9.—Aortic leaflet separation measurement (root function). The axes and abbreviations are the same as for Figure 3-4.

eccentric. Eccentricity probably is a function of echo beam angulation (Fig. 3-8).

Maximal aortic valve opening is measured in early systole from inner valve surface to inner valve surface (Fig. 3-2). Normal values are given in Table 3-5 and Figure 3-9. Aortic valves are thin and have very little inertia. This accounts for their abrupt opening and closure. Some values for normal valve opening velocity have been given for adults but no values are available for the pediatric patient.

Sweeping the transducer more cephalad causes the aortic cusps to be lost and the ascending aorta to be viewed. This maneuver is especially useful for examining patients with aortic stenosis and poststenotic aortic dilatation. Normally, the ascending aorta is equivalent in diameter to its root. Above the aortic valve, no landmark is present, so the precise location is not known.

LEFT ATRIUM

The cavity posterior to the aorta is the left atrium.[105] The measurement of left atrial dimension is made at the end of ventricular systole, i.e., as the aortic valve "box" closes, the left atrium is at its largest diameter. For standardization purposes, the measurement is made only in the plane that shows aortic valve leaflets (Figs. 3-1, 3-2 and 3-10).

The left atrial cavity is measured from the outside posterior aortic wall to the endocardial surface of the posterior left atrial wall. The posterior left atrial wall may appear quite ragged in places. The reason for this appearance is not known. When measuring the left atrial dimension, try to choose an area of the left atrial posterior wall that is smooth. Often, an inconsistent line is seen approximately three-fourths of the way posterior in the atrial cavity, which seems to have two walls (Fig. 3-10). Some investigators believe that this line repre-

Fig. 3-10.—Left atrial echocardiogram in a patient with patent ductus arteriosus, Z axis (**left**) and Y axis (**right**). This patient has increased left atrial cavity size. (Note the correlation of the left atrial size in the two axes.) The pertinent point to this figure, however, is the two-walled line demonstrated by the arrow in the left atrium in the left panel. This is a normal structure. See text for discussion. Abbreviations: *RVAW* = right ventricular anterior wall; *RVOT* = right ventricular outflow tract; *LAID* = left atrial internal dimension; *AO ARCH* = aortic arch; *RPA* = right pulmonary artery.

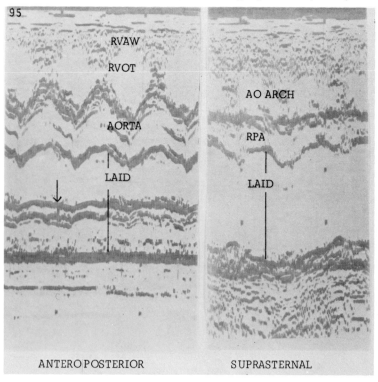

TABLE 3-6.—LEFT ATRIAL DIMENSION (END VENTRICULAR SYSTOLE) (IN CM)

(A) Neonates and Infants

	HAGAN	MEYER			SOLINGER			FEIGENBAUM
Weight	n = 200 m = 7.6 lb	n = 50 m = 3.2 kg	n = 21 2.27 kg	n = 28 2.73 kg	n = 25 3.18 kg	n = 22 3.64 kg	n = 23 4.09 kg	n = 26 0–25 lb m = 17 lb
Range	0.5–1.0	0.6–1.3	0.68–1.05	0.74–1.11	0.80–1.17	0.86–1.23	0.92–1.29	0.7–2.3
Mean	0.7 ± 0.01	0.9	0.87	0.93	0.99	1.05	1.11	1.7

(B) Older Children

	FEIGENBAUM				
Weight	n = 26 25–50 lb m = 39 lb	n = 20 50–75 lb m = 62 lb	n = 15 75–100 lb m = 89 lb	n = 11 100–125 lb m = 113 lb	n = 5 125–200 lb m = 165 lb
Range	1.7–2.7	1.9–2.8	2.0–3.0	2.1–3.0	2.1–3.7
Mean	2.2	2.3	2.4	2.7	2.8

sents pulmonary vein entry and others believe that it may be part of the posterior mitral annulus. Another possibility is that the atrial septum bulges into the left atrium and is transected by the beam. It could be a reflection or a phantom image. We believe that this line represents unfolded tissue of the anterior portion of the left atrial appendage. In any event, measurement of the left atrium must go deep to this line and to the true posterior left atrial wall.

We routinely examine patients through the suprasternal notch. An excellent study by B. Goldberg[81] showed that the sequence of structures encountered with this examination is the ascending aorta, the right pulmonary artery and the left atrium (Fig. 5-10). He confirmed this in cadavers, with angiography, and then applied it to a series of patients. Geometry of the left atrium can be fairly well ascertained by examining patients in both the Z and Y plane (via the precordial and suprasternal approaches). We have found that the left atrial dimension in the Y and Z coordinates is very similar in most patients (Figs. 3-10 and 5-11). These similar Y and Z measurements confirm that the left atrial shape is approximately spherical.

Table 3-6 and Figure 3-11 show normal values for left atrial dimension in the Z coordinate.

Fig. 3-11.—Precordial Z axis left atrial dimension measurement (root function). Axes and abbreviations are the same as for Figure 3-4. See text for details.

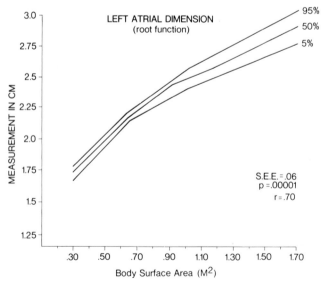

LEFT ATRIAL POSTERIOR WALL

The left atrial posterior wall is the next structure encountered by the beam (Figs. 3-1 and 3-2). The wall appears especially contractile as the beam approaches the mitral annulus (Figs. 3-1 and 5-7).

Posterior to the left atrial wall is the pericardium, then the pleura and the lung. The pericardium is very adherent to the left atrium because of the entrance of the pulmonary veins. Following the pericardial line from behind the left ventricle to behind the left atrium may help to identify the true left atrial posterior wall. It is a continuous line but it may not be a straight line, for the left atrium frequently dips posteriorly.

MITRAL VALVE

Leaving the aorta, as the transducer beam is angled caudad (Fig. 3-1), the anterior mitral valve leaflet is encountered. This valve is an important landmark for finding other cardiac structures. The diastolic motion has a characteristic M shape. The mitral valve has been said to have the greatest velocity of any cardiac structure but this is erro-

Fig. 3-12. — Diagram of the concept of multiple echoes. This figure shows the possibilities of valve intersection by ultrasound beams. The bottom line shows apposed valve leaflets encountered by the echo beam. This will be represented as a single line of closure. The middle line has four potential intersection sites. Multiple systolic lines would be expected. The top line shows the possibilities if the top of the valve leaflets were encountered. There should be two returning echoes in this instance. Angulation of the echo beam, from the bottom line to the top line, would bring about still further combinations and permutations. Eccentricity could also be induced.

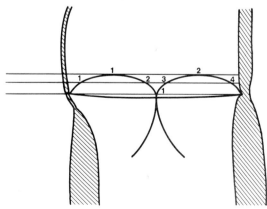

TABLE 3-7. – MITRAL VALVE DEPTH, AMPLITUDE AND VELOCITY (E-F SLOPE)

Neonates

	HAGAN	MEYER			SOLINGER		
Weight	n = 200 m = 7.6 lb	n = 50 m = 3.2 kg	n = 21 2.27 kg	n = 28 2.73 kg	n = 25 3.18 kg	n = 22 3.64 kg	n = 23 4.09 kg
Depth (cm)							
Range	—	3.1–4.7	—	—	—	—	—
Mean	—	3.8	—	—	—	—	—
Amplitude (cm)							
Range	0.60–1.20	0.6–1.2	.85–1.11	.89–1.15	.93–1.19	.97–1.23	1.01–1.27
Mean	0.81 ± 0.01	1.0	.98	1.02	1.06	1.10	1.14
Velocity (mm/sec)							
Range	60–130	38–80	—	—	—	—	—
Mean	80 ± 1	53	—	—	—	—	—

neous. The greatest velocity occurs in aortic valve opening. As the anterior mitral valve leaflet opens from point D, it moves toward the transducer and inscribes the first peak of the M—called the E point (Fig. 3-1). At this point, the anterior mitral valve leaflet may touch the septal surface. The valve then drifts posteriorly toward the closed position, either passively or because of papillary-chordae tightening during ventricular filling. Ventricular filling displaces the apex away from the valve ring. The farthest early point of posterior drift is the F point. Atrial contraction then forces the valve open again to the A point. The A generally is lower in amplitude than the E, although this can be variable in the abnormal. The valve then closes along the B slope to the C point. This is the most posterior point of the anterior mitral valve leaflet's late diastolic excursion.

The left ventricle moves anteriorly with systole as a unit and thus the line that represents the closed mitral leaflets moves anteriorly from the C point to the D point at the end of systole. The line of normal mitral closure frequently is not single, but may be multiple. These multiple echoes probably represent beam reflections from the multiple subtended surfaces of the mitral valve (Fig. 3-12). The same phenomenon can be seen during diastole for the same reason.

The velocity of the E—F slope of the mitral valve has been evaluated extensively in the adult. Normal ranges for children are given in Table 3-7. The most common use of this measurement is in evaluation of adult patients with mitral stenosis who demonstrate a decreased slope. It may be abnormally low in idiopathic hypertrophic subaortic stenosis, atrial septal defect and congestive cardiac failure. It may be abnormally high in mitral insufficiency or in other conditions causing rapid mitral flow. The E—F velocity is computed as a distance-time relationship, as shown in Figure 3-13.

The A—C interval is prolonged in congestive heart failure and in conditions associated with increased left ventricular end diastolic pressure.[56] It is receiving increasing attention in the adult patient and may have pediatric application as more work is done with it.

The anterior mitral valve depth is measured from the posterior chest wall to the C point. Amplitude is measured from the D point to the level of the E point in a perpendicular line (Figs. 3-2 and 3-13). Normal data are shown in Table 3-7 and Figure 3-14.

The D—E slope of the mitral opening is decreased in congestive cardiac failure with increased left ventricular end diastolic pressure.[56] Its slope is calculated by the right triangle method, as shown in Figure 3-13.

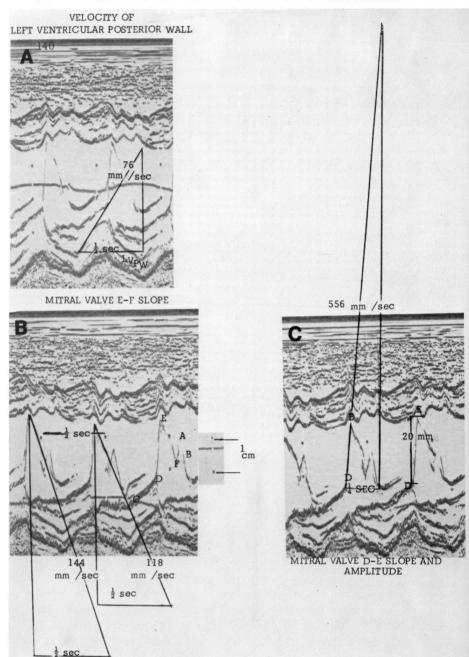

Fig. 3-13.—See legend on facing page.

TRANSITION AREA

As the echo beam passes through the anterior mitral valve leaflet it may strike the left atrial posterior wall or the left ventricular posterior wall. A helpful means of differentiating these structures is by observation of wall contraction in relation to electrocardiographic timing. Near the mitral annulus, the left atrial posterior wall moves anteriorly in middiastole and again after the electrocardiographic P wave (atrial systole) just before the electrocardiographic QRS. On the other hand, the left ventricular posterior wall moves anteriorly after the electrocardiographic QRS complex, in ventricular systole.

POSTERIOR MITRAL LEAFLET AND LEFT VENTRICLE

As the echocardiographic beam is directed more caudad (Fig. 3-2), the posterior mitral valve leaflet is seen simultaneously with the anterior mitral valve leaflet. It moves opposite to the anterior leaflet in a motion much like the clapping of hands. After the tip of the posterior mitral valve leaflet is recorded, the beam usually is in the left ventricular cavity. The farther the beam is directed posteriorly, leftward and inferiorly while viewing the posterior mitral leaflet the greater is

---

Fig. 3-13.—Velocity and amplitude measurements. Velocity measurements are made on the basis of right triangulation. Calibration markers are $\frac{1}{2}$ second apart in the X axis and 1 cm apart in the Y axis, permitting a distance-time relationship to be calculated. **A,** velocity of the left ventricular posterior wall contraction. A tangent is drawn along the slope of maximal contraction of the left ventricular posterior wall. A $\frac{1}{2}$-second base is drawn in the X axis from this tangent. A vertical line is drawn at the end of $\frac{1}{2}$ second intersecting the tangent. A tangent calibrated in millimeters then yields the velocity measurement, in this case 76 mm/sec. Note that the tangent has been multiplied by 2, as $\frac{1}{2}$ second was measured instead of 1 full second. **B,** the mitral valve E – F slope velocity has been calculated on two successive beats. A similar technique is used. A tangent is drawn along the E – F slope. A $\frac{1}{2}$-second line is inscribed in the X axis from the vertical line to the tangent. As $\frac{1}{2}$ second is used, the tangent is multipled by 2, yielding a value in the first beat of 144 mm/sec and a value in the second beat of 118 mm/sec. This example shows beat-to-beat variation of mitral valve velocity. The points of mitral valve motion are pictured in beat 3. **C,** calculation of mitral valve D – E slope velocity. In this case, a tangent is drawn from the D – E point. A line is drawn along the X axis, $\frac{1}{4}$ second from the D point. A vertical line is drawn perpendicular to the X axis, intersecting the tangent. The tangent then is measured. As $\frac{1}{4}$ second was used for the X axis, the value is multiplied by 4, yielding a D – E slope of 556 mm/sec. The D – E amplitude is measured in the next beat. Be sure to measure this in a perpendicular fashion rather than along the tangent. A value of 20 mm was obtained in this patient.

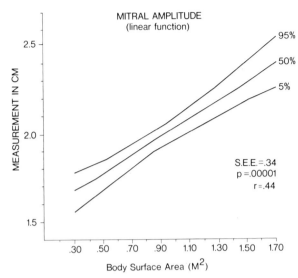

Fig. 3-14.—Mitral valve amplitude measurement (linear function). This function is measured from the D–E points of the mitral valve excursion (see Figs. 3-1, 3-2 and 3-13). See text for details. Axes and abbreviations are the same as for Figure 3-4.

the probability that the left ventricular wall is the posterior structure. As mentioned before, the left ventricle can be confirmed by observing the posterior wall contraction. The posterior left ventricular wall motion is anterior in systole and begins after the electrocardiographic QRS complex and slightly after septal contraction. The structure posterior to the mitral annulus must be evaluated cautiously, for it may be the atrial or the ventricular wall or a junctional area. Misinterpretation of the area will lead to erroneous measurements of wall thickness, ventricular cavity dimensions, Vcf and cardiac volumes.

LEFT VENTRICULAR POSTERIOR WALL

The layers of the left ventricular posterior wall include endocardium, myocardium and epicardium. Motion of the left ventricular posterior wall has been evaluated carefully by Jacobs[110] and by McDonald.[151] The left ventricular posterior wall excursion (amplitude) is measured perpendicularly from the maximal endocardial diastolic depth to the maximal systolic height (Figs. 3-2 and 3-13, C).

The left ventricular posterior wall contracts after the electrocardiographic QRS complex. Its contraction, along with septal contrac-

TABLE 3-8 (a).–LEFT VENTRICULAR POSTERIOR WALL THICKNESS (DIASTOLIC) (IN CM)

(A) Neonates and Infants

	HAGAN	SOLINGER					FEIGENBAUM
Weight	n = 200 m = 7.6 lb	n = 21 2.27 kg	n = 28 2.73 kg	n = 25 3.18 kg	n = 22 3.64 kg	n = 23 4.09 kg	n = 26 0 – 25 lb m = 17 lb
Range	.16 – .37	0.20 – 0.34	0.23 – 0.37	0.25 – 0.39	0.28 – 0.42	0.30 – 0.44	0.4 – 0.6
Mean	0.26 ± 0.001	0.27	0.30	0.32	0.35	0.37	0.5

(B) Older Children

	FEIGENBAUM				
Weight	n = 26 25 – 50 lb m = 39 lb	n = 20 50 – 75 lb m = 62 lb	n = 15 75 – 100 lb m = 89 lb	n = 11 100 – 125 lb m = 113 lb	n = 5 125 – 200 lb m = 165 lb
Range	0.5 – 0.7	0.6 – 0.7	0.7 – 0.8	0.7 – 0.8	0.7 – 0.8
Mean	0.6	0.7	0.7	0.7	0.8

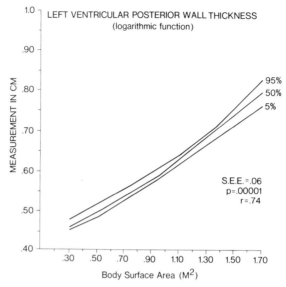

Fig. 3-15. — Left ventricular posterior wall thickness measurement (logarithmic function). See text for details. Axes and abbreviations are the same as for Figure 3-4.

tion, represents circumferential fiber shortening, which contributes to mitral valve closure and aortic valve opening. As blood is expelled and the ventricular cavities decrease in size, the heart becomes smaller. The left ventricular posterior wall amplitude represents a summation of the muscle contraction and cavity size decrease. Its amplitude thus is relatively greater than septal amplitude. Jacobs[110] showed that the normal adult value for mean left ventricular posterior wall amplitude is 1.2 cm and for mean septal amplitude is 0.5 cm.

Left ventricular posterior wall velocity is measured by the right triangle concept (Fig. 3-13).

Normal left ventricular posterior wall thickness data for children are shown in Table 3-8 (a) and Figure 3-15.

CARDIAC DEPTH

Cardiac depth is measured from the inside of the anterior chest wall to the pericardium at end diastole (Figs. 3-1 and 3-2). This measurement is useful for setting the depth control on the echocardiograph. Our data for cardiac depth are shown in Figure 3-16.

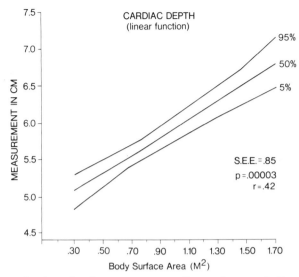

Fig. 3-16. — Cardiac depth measurement (linear function). See text for details. Axes and abbreviations are the same as for Figure 3-4.

SEPTAL DEPTH

Septal depth is measured from the inside of the anterior chest wall to the right septal surface (Figs. 3-1 and 3-2). This measurement is useful in adjusting the TGC and near gain controls on the echocardiograph.

Our normal data for septal depth are shown in Figure 3-17.

LEFT VENTRICULAR CAVITY AND FUNCTION

The left ventricular cavity is seen in panels 1 and 2 of Figure 3-1. As expected, it tapers toward the apex. The minor axis is in plane 2 just at the posterior mitral valve leaflet level. End diastolic and end systolic measurements are made only when the posterior mitral leaflet is seen. Normal data are shown in Tables 3-8 (b) and (c) and Figures 3-18 and 3-19.

Left ventricular volume and ejection fraction have been estimated by echocardiography. The estimation of left ventricular volume from single plane dimensions assumes that the left ventricular cavity is a predictable shape and that there is a standard relationship between the major and minor axes of the left ventricular cavity over the range of ventricular volumes. Further, it is assumed that the left ventricle

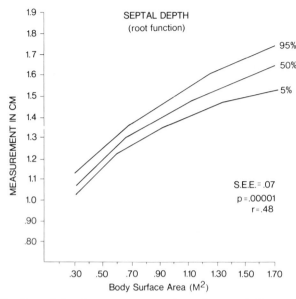

Fig. 3-17. — Septal depth measurement (root function). See text for details. Axes and abbreviations are the same as for Figure 3-4.

is an ellipsoid of revolution whose semi-minor axes are equal and are approximately one-half the length of the semi-major axis. Therefore, the formula for the calculation of the volume of an ellipsoid is

$$V = \frac{\pi}{6} \times D_1 \times D_2 \times L \qquad (3.1)$$

where D_1 and D_2 are the semi-minor axes and L is the semi-major axis.

$$\text{If } D_1 = D_2, \text{ then } V = \frac{\pi}{6} D^2 L \qquad (3.2)$$

If the semi-major axis is assumed to be twice the semi-minor axes, the formula may be further simplified to

$$V = \frac{\pi}{6} D^2 \times 2D \qquad (3.3)$$

or

$$V = \frac{\pi}{3} D^3 \qquad (3.4)$$

Since $\frac{\pi}{3}$ is approximate unity, a further approximation can be made:

$$V = D^3 \qquad (3.5)$$

TABLE 3-8 (b). – LEFT VENTRICULAR END DIASTOLIC DIMENSION (IN CM)
(A) Neonates and Infants

	HAGAN	MEYER		SOLINGER				FEIGENBAUM
Weight	n = 200 m = 7.6 lb	n = 50 m = 3.2 kg	n = 21 2.27 kg	n = 28 2.73 kg	n = 25 3.18 kg	n = 22 3.64 kg	n = 23 4.09 kg	n = 26 0 – 25 lb m = 17 lb
Range	1.20 – 2.33	1.2 – 2.0	1.61 – 2.17	1.65 – 2.21	1.70 – 2.26	1.75 – 2.31	1.80 – 2.36	1.3 – 3.2
Mean	1.87 ± 0.03	1.6	1.89	1.93	1.98	2.03	2.08	2.4

(B) Older Children

FEIGENBAUM

Weight	n = 26 25 – 50 lb m = 39 lb	n = 20 50 – 75 lb m = 62 lb	n = 15 75 – 100 lb m = 89 lb	n = 11 100 – 125 lb m = 113 lb	n = 5 125 – 200 lb m = 165 lb
Range	2.4 – 3.8	3.3 – 4.5	3.5 – 4.7	3.7 – 4.9	4.4 – 5.2
Mean	3.4	3.8	4.1	4.3	4.9

TABLE 3-8 (c). – LEFT VENTRICULAR END
SYSTOLIC DIMENSION (IN CM)
Neonates

	HAGAN
	n = 200 m = 7.6 lb
Weight	
Range	0.80 – 1.86
Mean	1.33 ± 0.03

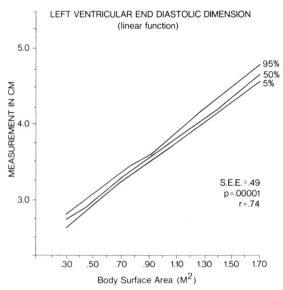

Fig. 3-18.—Left ventricular cavity, end diastolic measurement (linear function). See text for details. Axes and abbreviations are the same as for Figure 3-4.

Fig. 3-19.—Left ventricular cavity, end systolic measurement (root function). See text for details. Axes and abbreviations are the same as for Figure 3-4.

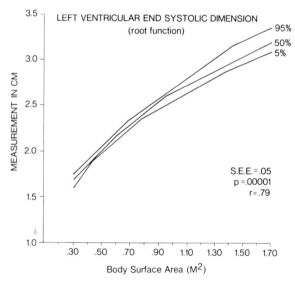

Although these assumptions have led to volume calculations with reasonable correlation to other techniques in adults,[10, 71, 74, 177, 182, 186] the correlation of echo and angio volume has been less acceptable in children.[156] It must be recognized that the calculation of chamber volume from a cube function of a single diastolic or systolic dimension entails cubing of any error in that measurement. The inability to exactly transect the ventricle in the minor axis is an angulation error. The angular errors involved in studying left ventricular dimensions in small children or newborns has, in our experience, led to prohibitively large errors in volume calculations. Nevertheless, Meyer *et al.*[156] calculated left ventricular volume in children from single crystal dimensions and correlated the study with biplane left ventricular angiography. A regression equation was derived to allow estimation of volume directly from end diastolic and/or systolic left ventricular dimensions.

Fortuin *et al.*[71] found that the volume formula (3.5) was correct until left ventricular volume dilatation occurred, changing the chamber from a prolate ellipse to a spherical shape. Their regression equations are:

$$ESV = 47\, S_{s\,echo} - 120$$

and

$$EDV = 59\, S_{d\,echo} - 153$$

where $S_{s\,echo}$ = end systolic dimension and $S_{d\,echo}$ = end diastolic dimension.

Obviously, volumes may be calculated for systole and for diastole. The difference between the two volumes (*EDV* and *ESV*) is stroke volume. Stroke volume divided by end diastolic volume is ejection fraction. Popp and Harrison[182] used a model of a geometric prolate ellipse and developed a regression equation of

$$SV = 1.047\, (Dd^3 - Ds^3)$$

where *SV* = stroke volume, *Dd* = diastolic dimension and *Ds* = systolic dimension.

The mean velocity of circumferential fiber shortening (mean Vcf) is an expression of cardiac muscle function that describes the fractional degree of shortening of a theoretic circumferential muscle fiber, related to the time during which the shortening occurs, and is expressed by the formula

Vcf (expressed in circumferences per sec)

$$= \frac{\text{end diastolic dimension (mm)} - \text{end systolic dimension (mm)}}{\text{end diastolic dimension (mm)} \times \text{ejection time (sec)}} \quad (3.6)$$

Previous studies[30, 173] in adults have shown excellent correlation of mean Vcf and left ventricular function parameters measured invasively. Patients with and without ventricular muscle disease were identified by this parameter. Since mean Vcf is normalized for end diastolic dimension and involves no power function, it is significantly less prone to error from minor dimensional discrepancies. In our experience, values for the mean Vcf obtained from slightly different areas of the midportion of the same ventricle are essentially identical and highly reproducible. Despite its sensitivity to changes in afterload (the resistance against which the ventricle must eject blood), the index is useful both as a parameter of cardiac muscle function and as an estimation of the ejection work performed by the left ventricle. In situations in which afterload is stable, serial measurements pertain more to muscle function than to ejection work. However, in the presence of left-to-right shunts with a low-resistance lung circulation, the index is useful for estimating shunt size. The following discussion summarizes our experience with mean Vcf as a left ventricular function parameter.[195]

Left ventricular diastolic and systolic dimension were measured at the site of maximal excursion, which was identified by sweeping the left ventricle from body to outflow tract. Preliminary studies using a phased multicrystal system for cross-sectional imaging suggested that the mitral leaflet in children hangs farther into the left ventricle than in adults. Therefore, we consider that appropriate measures of left ventricular posterior wall and septal motion are obtained in the plane of maximal mitral excursion. The mitral valve was used for timing purposes to identify end diastole and end systole. Ejection time was measured from the point of complete mitral valve closure to the onset of mitral valve opening. These points correspond closely to the onset and termination of left ventricular systolic wall motion and are easily identified. No correction was applied for the pre-ejection period, as the values for ejection time in our initial infant studies were almost identical to those reported in normal infants by axillary artery tracings.[139] Values for mean Vcf were calculated according to formula 3.6.

Initial studies comparing mean Vcf determinations obtained by sequential ultrasound and cineangiographic methods in children with heart disease showed a correlation coefficient of +0.97 and attested to the reliability of the ultrasound-derived index. Mean Vcf data for a group of normal newborn infants of various ages had a mean of 1.51 ± 0.04 (SE) circumferences/sec. There were no statistical differences between the age subgroups in the newborn period. Serial studies performed in normal newborns revealed no substantial changes within the newborn period after age 10 hours.

The group mean for Vcf for 45 older children without cardiac abnormality between ages 5 and 15 was 1.34 ± 0.03 (SE).

CHORDAE TENDINEAE

In the area just caudad to the posterior mitral valve leaflet, several thin lines can be found near the posterior left ventricular wall. These represent chordae tendineae and attach the posterior mitral valve leaflet to the papillary muscles. Sometimes these are confused with endocardial echoes and must be recognized as a different structure. One reason for confusion is that chordae move parallel to the posterior left ventricular wall. This is due to their close relationship to the wall (Fig. 3-1). Correct identification often is possible by following the posterior left ventricular wall throughout the sweep (Figs. 3-1 and 5-6).

PAPILLARY MUSCLES

The chordae terminate in papillary muscles. These muscles are located apically and contract during systole (Figs. 3-1 and 5-6). Avoid this area of the ventricle when evaluating septal motion, cavity size or posterior left ventricular wall thickness. This area should be evaluated for an aneurysm, diverticulum or abnormally contracting muscle.

PERICARDIUM

The next posterior structure in the echo path is the pericardium, which usually is seen as a heavy line. The epi- and pericardium usually form a single line. The posterior pericardial reflection is fixed to the left atrium and pulmonary veins, but it still is a continuous structure from the area behind the left ventricle to the area behind the left atrium.

PLEURA AND LUNG

Posterior to the pericardium is the pleura and deep to that is the lung. No structures can be imaged behind the lung. Often, if the cardiac echo is compressed on the record, parallel moving lines can be seen in the lung that seem to represent the posterior thoracic aorta.

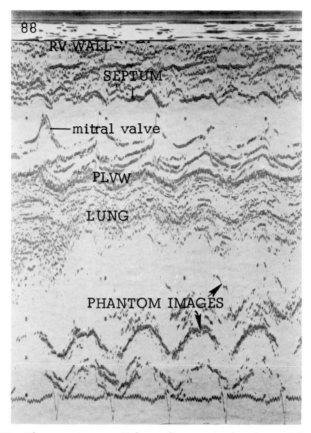

Fig. 3-20. — Phantom images. Echocardiogram in the plane of the posterior mitral valve leaflet. Note the images posterior to the pericardium in the area of the lung. The two phantom images labeled with arrows appear as valves. Just above the electrocardiogram is another phantom that resembles the ventricular wall or aorta. Abbreviations: *RV Wall* = right ventricular anterior wall; *PLVW* = posterior left ventricular wall.

These lines are not the posterior descending aorta, but are reflections or "phantom" re-echoes (Fig. 3-20).

TRICUSPID VALVE

The tricuspid valve has a movement similar to that of the mitral valve. Amplitude and velocity measurement techniques are similar to those for the mitral valve. Velocity values have been computed for this valve and are slower than for the mitral. Normal data are presented in Table 3-9 and Figure 3-21. It is necessary to view the valve

TABLE 3-9.—TRICUSPID VALVE DEPTH, AMPLITUDE AND VELOCITY (E-F SLOPE)
(*Neonates*)

	HAGAN	MEYER	SOLINGER				
Weight	n = 200 m = 7.6 lb	n = 50 m = 3.2 kg	n = 21 2.27 kg	n = 28 2.73 kg	n = 25 3.18 kg	n = 22 3.64 kg	n = 23 4.09 kg
Depth (cm)							
Range	—	2.4–3.2	—	—	—	—	—
Mean	—	2.8	—	—	—	—	—
Amplitude (cm)							
Range	0.70–1.40	0.8–1.4	0.88–1.2	0.92–1.24	0.97–1.29	1.01–1.33	1.06–1.38
Mean	0.93 ± 0.02	1.1	1.04	1.08	1.13	1.17	1.22
Velocity (mm/sec)							
Range	60–116	34–56	—	—	—	—	—
Mean	93 ± 2	43	—	—	—	—	—

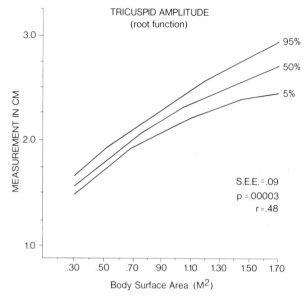

Fig. 3-21.—Tricuspid valve amplitude measurement (root function). See text for details. Axes and abbreviations are the same as for Figure 3-4.

during every echocardiographic examination to rule out tricuspid stenosis and tricuspid atresia. The tricuspid valve is found easily in normal children (Fig. 5-5) but is more difficult to view in the adult.

The tricuspid valve is not continuous with the aorta, as septum is interspersed between it and the aorta. However, an echocardiographic relationship occasionally is referred to as "tricuspid-aortic continuity." Because of the interspersed septal tissue, this is *not* an actual continuity.

RIGHT ATRIUM

To date, little success has been achieved with echocardiographic evaluation of the right atrium. Its shape is irregular and it often lies substernally and under an area of the right lung. Much work remains to be done with this chamber.

PULMONARY VALVE

The pulmonary valve usually is difficult to see in adults but it nearly always is possible to record in children. We recorded it in 90% of normal examinations. The pulmonary valve opens just after the QRS complex (Fig. 3-2). Weyman *et al.*[233] and Gramiak *et al.*[89] have shown,

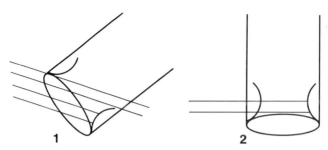

Fig. 3-22. — Diagrammatic representation of the effect of angulation of the pulmonary artery on the echo beam passage. In the first panel, the pulmonary artery is diagrammed as it is viewed in the lateral plane, angling backward. The echo beam will strike the posterior pulmonary valve perpendicularly but will be more parallel to the anterior pulmonary valve. This anterior valve reflection will ricochet toward the upper part of the body and the echo would not be sensed by the transducer. This explains why only the echo of the posterior pulmonary valve was observed in the first panel in Figure 3-2. Note also that the anterior pulmonary root may reflect the echo beam but the measurement from anterior to posterior root will give a larger pulmonary root measurement than a true cross section. This is an elliptical section. In the second panel, the pulmonary artery arises perpendicularly from the heart. In this instance, both pulmonary valves will be seen and accurate pulmonary root measurements can be made. This situation is unusual in older children.

and we concur, that the pulmonary valve may open as the result of right atrial contraction before ventricular systole begins. The valve then drifts toward closure and is reopened by ventricular systole.

We cannot always visualize the boxlike cusp motion of the pulmonary valve because the pulmonary artery exits from the heart somewhat posteriorly rather than vertically. Thus, only the posterior leaflet of the pulmonary valve is viewed. The anterior leaflet is primarily parallel to the echo beam and these echoes accordingly will not be sensed by the transducer (Fig. 3-22). Sometimes both walls of the pulmonary artery are recorded and measurements can be made. When both the leaflets are observed, the interpulmonic cusp distance can be measured. Typical patterns of pulmonary valve motion are shown in Figures 3-2 and 5-9.

RATIOS

Some coincidental and teleologic measurement relationships exist and are handy when evaluating echocardiograms. These include the ratios of the left atrium to the aorta, and the septum to the left ventricular posterior wall. The ratios are not age or body size related except in the premature and neonate. Beyond this age, the left atrial

TABLE 3-10. — RATIOS

	PERCENTILE		
	5%	50%	95%
Left atrium/aorta	0.84	1.04	1.28
Septum/left ventricular posterior wall	0.75	1.00	1.23

No correlation to body surface area.

dimension approximately equals the aortic root diameter and the septal thickness approximately equals left ventricular posterior wall thickness. In the premature, the aortic root may grossly exceed the left atrial dimension and the septal thickness may exceed the left ventricular posterior wall thickness. With growth, our premature and neonatal patients with these unusual ratios have progressed to normal ratios.

Normal ratios of left atrium to aorta, and septum to left ventricular posterior wall in our 100 patients are shown in Table 3-10.

Chapter 4 deals with echocardiographic evaluation of some congenital cardiac abnormalities.

4 / The Abnormal Echocardiogram

INTRODUCTORY STATEMENT

PEDIATRIC ECHOCARDIOGRAPHY clearly is in its early stages. Not all lesions have been studied, and the final word is not yet available for those that have been investigated recently. However, a similar state-of-the-art is true in many fields of medicine, and this fact should not preclude a compilation of the knowledge available to date. Unfortunately, not all known information has been published, and that which *is* published may not appear in critically reviewed journals. Some data are available only in abstract form or in the form of personal communication.

The purpose of this chapter is to acquaint the reader with the presently available information and to provide adequate referencing to permit perusal of the original work. The authors will comment on their experience with lesions in order to relate problems that have been encountered with regard to "diagnostic criteria." Any of our observations that may be pertinent will be added. We have made a practice of attempting to validate the work of others to the maximal extent possible. Additionally, we evaluated normal children to see if the diagnostic criteria for lesions occurred and which false positives exist in a normal population. In many instances, we have been able to corroborate the work of others, but in some instances we have not. In all instances, we will attempt to provide the reader with echocardiographic material to demonstrate all points of view. If enough data are available, the reader is urged to form his own opinion.

4.1. Atrial Secundum Defect

Pertinent literature references: 11, 37, 98, 115, 120, 145, 149, 155, 186, 211, 218, 219, 221, 222, 223, 227.

Review of Published Information:

The atrial septal defect has been studied extensively by echocardiography. The most commonly recognized features of this defect are that:

1. Ventricular septal motion usually is paradoxical with respect to normal.

2. The right ventricle is dilated.

Paradoxical Septal Motion:

Normally, the ventricular septum moves posteriorly in systole.[37]

The effect of this motion is to constrict the left ventricle. Accordingly, in the normal, the septum does not constrict the right ventricle but action of the anterior right ventricular wall and movement of the heart as a whole does. Paradoxical septal motion (anterior systolic septal motion) occurs in pathologic situations in which significant right ventricular volume overload (RVVO) is present. Therefore, tricuspid insufficiency, pulmonary insufficiency, atrial septal defects and total anomalous pulmonary venous return may cause this abnormality. Paradoxical septal motion has also been observed in complete left bundle-branch block. Paradoxical septal motion has been experimentally induced acutely when the right ventricle was overloaded and was reversed when the acute experimental overload was removed.[43] Left ventricular function in patients with right ventricular overload may be altered because the septum moves away from the left ventricular posterior wall during contraction.

The Echo Demonstration:

Demonstration of paradoxical septal motion is neither simple nor always possible in right ventricular volume overload.[223] False positives may arise because the top of the normal ventricular septum is tethered to the aorta. Therefore, the normal upper septum always moves "paradoxically," since the aorta moves anteriorly with systole, dragging this portion of the septum along with it. The bottom of the normal left ventricular septum always moves to constrict the left ventricle. Thus, in the normal heart, septal motion is a complex hinged action with the fulcrum usually high, near the aorta. With right ventricular volume overload, the pivot point is shifted lower in the septum.[98] For this reason, it is necessary to record the midportion of the septum in the plane of the posterior mitral valve leaflet when looking for paradoxical septal motion.

Two types of abnormal septal motion have been described in right ventricular volume overload.[37] The most common is Type A,[37, 149] in which the midseptum moves anteriorly in systole and posteriorly in diastole (Fig. 4-1). Thus, septal motion parallels the motion of the left ventricular posterior wall. Type B motion is defined as flat septal motion with slight posterior motion in early diastole (Fig. 4-2). Many of the recordings demonstrating Type B septal motion may have been obtained in the region of a displaced hinge point. Flat septal motion, which looks like Type B, can also occur in septal infarction,[110] but this problem is uncommon in children.

The paradoxical septal motion of right ventricular volume overload usually disappears within several weeks to months postoperatively.[155]

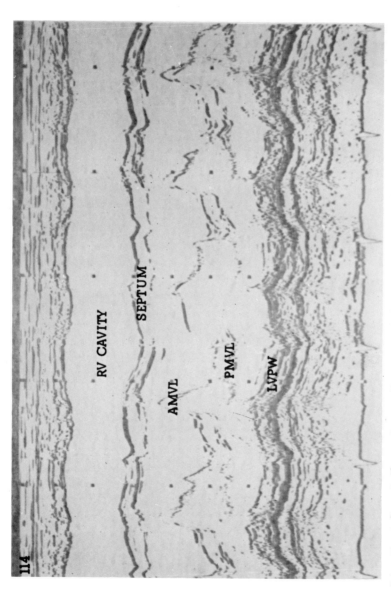

Fig. 4-1.—Example of Type A paradoxical septal motion in atrial septal defect. The septum moves principally anteriorly after the QRS complex. The right ventricular cavity is dilated. The anterior right ventricular wall is thickened because the patient had pulmonary stenosis in addition to the atrial septal defect.

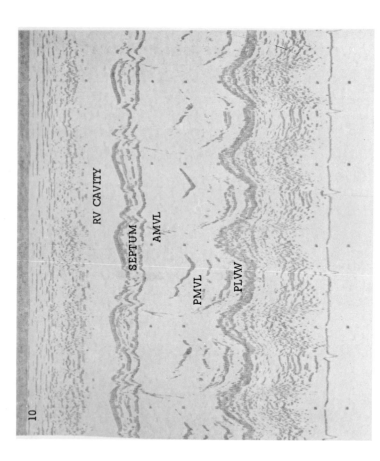

Fig. 4-2.—Type B paradoxical septal motion. Septal motion is mainly flat in this patient with atrial septal defect. Slight septal posterior motion occurs near the end of systole. Right ventricular septal motion is clearly anterior during systole. The right ventricular wall is not well shown in this example, but the cavity is relatively large. The right side of the septum constricts the right ventricular cavity during systole.

Right Ventricular Dilatation:

Right ventricular volume overload should cause the right ventricular cavity to be dilated. In patients with right ventricular volume overload, the right ventricular cavity dimension usually approaches that of the left ventricle. Failure to demonstrate increased right ventricular dimension should arouse suspicion regarding the presence of or extent of right ventricular volume overload.

Observations about Atrioventricular Valves with Right Ventricular Volume Overload:

Kamigaki and Goldschlager[120] noted significantly decreased D–E slopes of the anterior and posterior mitral leaflets in patients with atrial septal defects. This probably is due to the dynamics of the lesion, which allows flow from the left to the right atrium as well as normal forward flow. Thus, the left atrium has already partially decompressed before the mitral valve opens. Ultan et al.[227] measured the "slope of the E wave," which probably is the E–F slope, and indicated that it was normal in patients with secundum defects. They suggest that the tricuspid valve slope was increased.

Other abnormalities of the mitral valve have been noted. Tajik et al.[222] reported "pseudo-IHSS" in a patient with atrial secundum defect. In this patient, mitral systolic anterior motion was noted. In an angiographic study, Betriu et al.[11] reported that 37% of patients with atrial secundum defects had prolapse of the posterior mitral leaflet. This interesting observation has, in our experience, been substantiated by echocardiography.

Our Experience with This Diagnosis:

Right ventricular volume overload usually can be diagnosed in patients with significant left-to-right shunts or pulmonary insufficiency. We have failed to demonstrate paradoxical septal motion in patients with small atrial septal defects, mild to moderate pulmonary insufficiency and in some patients with tricuspid insufficiency. Additionally, we have observed 2 children with large left-to-right shunts who repeatedly had normal septal motion. Both had increased right ventricular dimension. In several patients, the right ventricular dimension has been less than half that of the left ventricular dimension when measured in the plane of the posterior mitral valve leaflet.

The ease with which the diagnosis of right ventricular volume overload is made is variable. Paradoxical septal motion can be relatively simple to record in some patients and very difficult and time consuming to find in others. We would like to offer two additional comments to bear in mind during evaluation of patients with these conditions.

In contrast to the electrocardiographic finding of "hypertrophy," true right ventricular anterior wall thickening is rare in children, for they rarely have pulmonary vascular obstructive disease with isolated secundum atrial septal defects. The electrocardiographic hypertrophy may represent right ventricular dilatation. If significant right ventricular wall thickening is present with signs of right ventricular volume overload, the examiner should consider a complex lesion. We have not found a patient with gross anterior right ventricular wall hypertrophy accompanying an isolated atrial septal defect. However, a thick anterior right ventricular wall may accompany pulmonary insufficiency in a patient with a repaired pulmonary outflow tract if the hypertrophy has remained unresolved.

The left atrium usually is of normal size in patients with simple secundum atrial septal defects. In children, blood from the left atrium passes into the right atrium because right ventricular compliance almost always is greater than left ventricular compliance. Thus, a large left atrium should arouse suspicion about the diagnosis of isolated secundum atrial defect.

Points of Caution:

1. Do not consider that all patients with paradoxical septal motion have atrial septal defects, for this finding accompanies the generic condition of right ventricular volume overload.

2. The septum must be recorded in its midportion. This is ensured most often by simultaneous recording of the posterior mitral valve leaflet. Recording the septum too high or too low can give erroneous results. It is best to study the whole septum.

3. Record both sides of the septal wall simultaneously as well as the left ventricular posterior and right ventricular anterior walls.

4. Remember that a few patients with right ventricular volume overload do not exhibit all classic findings.

5. Flat septal motion (Type B) may be due to septal infarction. The latter may be associated with increased right ventricular cavity dimension.

6. Left bundle-branch block affects septal motion and may cause confusion (see section 4.31).

7. Some complex lesions can cause aberrations of usual findings. Consider, for example, a patient with a left-to-right shunt through an atrial septal defect who also has a single ventricle.

8. Mitral systolic closure may resemble systolic anterior motion without IHSS in the presence of right ventricular volume overload (see section 4.10).

9. A decreased D–E or E–F slope of the mitral valve may be present.

4.2. Patent Ductus Arteriosus

Patent ductus arteriosus is a common neonatal lesion. Infants with respiratory distress often have this lesion, and the left-to-right shunt through it may be very large. If an infant has respiratory distress syndrome, he already has tachypnea and tachycardia. The chest x-ray often has such parenchymal changes that the heart is obscured. The liver may descend because of lung hyperinflation if he is on a ventilator. This makes assessment of congestive failure difficult. Cardiac catheterization can be done but assessment of shunt size is difficult because mixing of arterialized and venous blood is limited. Pulmonary arteriography can be done and the levophase will allow measurement of left atrial size to indirectly quantitate small, moderate or large shunts.

Because the site of the ductus arteriosus cannot be visualized, no primary echocardiographic diagnosis is possible. However, secondary characteristics, such as enlarged left atrium and left ventricle, are present, but these characteristics are similar to the secondary ones for ventricular septal defect. No reports of echocardiographic diagnosis of this lesion have appeared in the literature.

Our Experience with This Lesion:

We have had considerable experience with echocardiography of patients with patent ductus arteriosus. We record echocardiograms for all children with respiratory distress syndrome treated with assisted ventilation in order to follow left atrial size. This chamber dimension is a sensitive way of following the magnitude of the left-to-right shunt through the patent ductus. Additionally, the echocardiogram can rule out some other types of cardiac problems. Serial left atrial dimensions are recorded in these children and change in size of the left atrium is charted. Infants weighing between 900 and 1300 grams have a smaller left atrial than aortic dimension. The left atrium normally ranges from about 4 to 5 mm. For infants between 1300 and 2000 grams, left atrial dimension varies from 5 to 9 mm. Children from approximately 2000 to 3000 grams have normal left atrial dimension of 9–12 mm. Those in the smallest weight group, in our experience, have been able to tolerate left-to-right shunts that distend their left atrium to about 9 mm. Children in the middle size group seem to tolerate left atrial dimensions smaller than 14 mm and those in the largest group tolerate about 17 mm. These are generalizations, but they have been quite useful. It is clear that left atrial size must be followed frequently, for it can increase or decrease quickly. We have observed 82 children, many of whom were very symptomatic and had large left atria. Some of these children have had spontaneous ductal closure and demonstrated a decrease in left atrial size. Others have required ligation of the patent ductus. These ductus were of the same external dimension as the aorta. They were thin walled and thus had very significant internal diameters. No pattern is obvious other than the association of symptomatology and left atrial size. In our experience, the pulse pressure, the intensity of the murmur, presence of diastolic murmurs and electrocardiograms have been far less sensitive indices than the left atrial dimension for predicting changes in the shunt size.

In small premature infants it may be useful to express left atrial size as a left atrial/aortic ratio that assists in, but does not solve, normalization. This ratio is a predictor of shunt size. In 110 normal term and premature infants, left atrial/aortic ratio was 0.741 ± 0.13 (S.D.). In patients with large patent ductus arteriosus (n = 83), left atrial/aortic ratio was 1.19 ± 0.18 (S.D.). These differences were statistically significant ($p < 0.001$). Finally, the patterns of wall-to-septal motion expressed as mean Vcf have also been used as a predictor of shunt size.

Serial studies of a single patient are most useful for considering surgical intervention. As the effects of cardiac and respiratory disease are difficult to separate in these critically ill premature infants, non-invasive assessment of shunt size is very advantageous.

Points of Caution:

1. The left atrial size above which children seem to have severe problems with patent ductus arteriosus left-to-right shunt is a generalization, and some latitude exists for a given child. Charting left atrial dimension frequently is much more important than measuring a left atrial size once. Obviously, an increase in symptomatology or a rapidly increasing left atrial dimension cannot be ignored. Normalization by measuring left atrial/aortic ratio may be of assistance.

2. Some children with respiratory distress syndrome have severe sternal retraction and this flattens the left atrium. A suprasternal notch left atrial assessment is imperative in these children. On occasion, we have lifted the sternum with a suture to make the precordial (Z) (left atrial) measurement. The left atrial Z size can change dramatically with this maneuver.

3. Children with patent ductus arteriosus may have other cardiac lesions. An echocardiogram may or may not reveal these. Complete

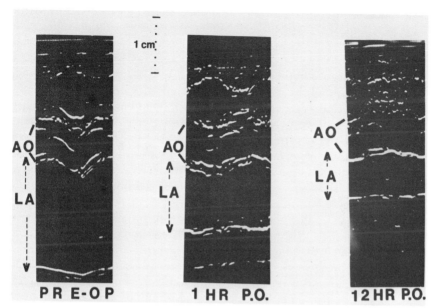

Fig. 4-3.—Ductus ligation. Three Polaroid echocardiograms from the same child are shown. Instrument settings were not changed in order to keep the calibration precisely similar. The left atrium in the left-hand panel, immediately before surgery, is slightly larger than 2 cm. The child had surgery and as soon as he was resituated in the intensive care unit, approximately 1 hour following the actual ligation of the ductus, the left atrium had already decreased to about 1.2 cm. Twelve hours after ligation, the left atrium was about 0.8 cm. The aortic size remained unchanged. The aortic valve is demonstrated in each panel. Arrows refer to the left atrial internal dimension.

cardiac care and examination are essential; do not rely only on the echocardiogram.

4. The left atrial dimension will mirror changes in pulmonary blood flow. These changes in pulmonary blood flow are not necessarily solely related to left-to-right shunt. For example, the left atrium may be increased because of hypervolemia, acidosis, hypoxia or bradycardia. The last three decrease myocardial contractility and require a higher filling pressure of the left ventricle.

5. Left atrial dimension may decrease markedly with digitalis or diuresis only to increase again in 4–6 hours as the shunt becomes larger. One period of improvement in the left atrial dimension does not necessarily signal an end to the problem.

6. Be certain that the left atrial dimension is measured to the back wall of the left atrium and that the echo is of good technical quality,

as decisions are made on the basis of a change of a few millimeters.

7. Left atrial dimension usually decreases markedly postoperatively (Fig. 4-3).

4.3. Ventricular Septal Defect

Pertinent literature references: 19, 56, 89, 130, 158, 211, 227.

Ventricular septal defect is the most common cardiac anomaly. This lesion may occur as an isolated entity or in combination with other lesions. This section will treat only the isolated type. The site and size of the defect may vary, and therefore the lesion has a broad pathologic spectrum. At first glance, it might seem that the lesion is ideally suited for primary diagnosis by echocardiography. It would be predicted that the beam could be directed through the defect and demonstrate the absence of part of the septum and the presence of the remainder. Unfortunately, this rarely is the case. Several practical factors must be considered to understand the nature of the problem. First, the normal septum may not always be viewed easily because the angle between the septum and the transducer may not be 90°. This would produce apparent absence of the septum even though it were present. Even more perplexing is the problem of slight septal rotation with each beat in some children. This causes the septum to be perpendicular to the beam during some of the cardiac cycle and at a different angle at other parts of the cycle. This rotational phenomenon causes the normal septum to appear to be broken. It is impossible to know if the septum is intact but rotating around the perpendicular or if a defect exists. Second, ultrasonic beam width may be large with respect to defect size (Fig. 4-4). This would tend to obscure the defect and make the septum appear whole. Finally, the defect edges may overlap in the plane of examination. In this instance, the viewer would always see septum and not recognize the slitlike defect (Fig. 4-4).

Occasionally large ventricular septal defects can be observed by single crystal echocardiography. Most commonly, these are found as:

1. An area in which the tricuspid and mitral valve can be visualized but no septum is present, or

2. An area in which the septum repeatedly drops out during a sweep from the septal surface to the aortic wall.

The easiest ventricular septal defect to demonstrate by echocardiography occurs in tetralogy of Fallot, which is covered elsewhere in this chapter.

Despite the frequent occurrence of ventricular septal defect, it has attracted little attention in the echocardiographic literature. Most

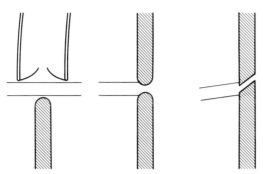

Fig. 4-4.—Echocardiography of a ventricular septal defect. In the right-hand panel, the very small ventricular septal defect is shown as a slit. The echo beam probably will not find this particular type of ventricular septal defect, for the beam always subtends some portion of muscle. In the center panel, the beam is relatively large with respect to the ventricular septal defect. This defect may or may not be found by echocardiography. One must also remember that the septum is in motion, and that this complicates identification. In the left-hand panel, the beam clearly passes below the aortic cusps and misses the septum entirely. This is the situation with tetralogy of Fallot. This defect probably will be found by echocardiography.

often, cases of ventricular septal defect have been used as controls for other studies or have appeared in lists of defects that have been observed by echocardiography.[158, 211] Ultan et al.[227] suggested that high mitral valve flow in ventricular septal defect and other conditions causes rapid valve velocity. Ventricular septal defects have been observed by "B" scan gating techniques.[130]

Secondary detection, i.e., observing the effects of the defect, is considerably easier than primary detection. Large ventricular septal defects in patients with no pulmonary vascular obstructive disease cause increased pulmonary blood flow. This increased pulmonary blood flow returns to the left side of the heart and causes dilatation of the left atrium and left ventricle. The right ventricular anterior wall usually is of normal thickness and the right ventricular cavity is of normal size or only slightly enlarged. Left ventricular wall thickness almost invariably is normal. Septal and left ventricular posterior wall motion may be increased in response to the high volume ejection. The direction of septal motion is normal. If a right-to-left shunt is present, right ventricular anterior wall thickness is increased, left atrial size is decreased and left ventricular dimension may be decreased. If pulmonary vascular obstructive disease is present, diastolic pulmonary valve motion is flat.[89] Unfortunately, none of these findings separates a ventricular septal defect from a patent ductus arteriosus, but the differentiation can be made clinically.

Our Experience with This Lesion:

Echocardiography is very useful in following patients with ventricular septal defect. We rarely can make an echocardiographic primary diagnosis by recording absence of a part of the septum. Furthermore, we rarely can pinpoint the location of the defect. Secondary signs are more useful.

Shunt flow correlates well with left atrial size.[19] We routinely chart left atrial size to observe for increasing shunt flows. We regard any sudden left atrial expansion in an infant as a warning sign of impending congestive cardiac failure.

Left atrial size should be evaluated in two coordinates, Y and Z. This is achieved by recording a precordial and a suprasternal echocardiogram. Use of two coordinates helps to eliminate the possibility that the left atrium may be flattened or otherwise misshapen. Left ventricular size is helpful but to a lesser extent than left atrial size. The pattern of exaggerated septal and posterior wall motion in patients with large left-to-right shunts has been associated with increased Vcf. If the left-to-right shunt is large and cardiac function is normal, Vcf will mirror the shunt size.

We regard any increase in right ventricular anterior wall thickness as suggestive of potential pulmonary vascular obstructive disease or pulmonary stenosis. Left ventricular wall thickness rarely is increased in the isolated ventricular septal defect despite the frequent electrocardiographic interpretation of "left ventricular hypertrophy" in this lesion. Those patients with true left ventricular posterior wall thickening usually have had a coarctation of the aorta or aortic stenosis in addition to the ventricular septal defect.

Small pericardial effusions are very common in patients with left-to-right shunts and should not be viewed with undue alarm.

Postoperatively, it is fairly common to observe the patch covering the ventricular septal defect, but the technique is particularly insensitive for making the diagnosis of patch separation postoperatively.

Points of Caution:

1. Do not often expect to see the ventricular septal defect as a "hole" in the septal echo.

2. Judgment of left atrial size requires a two-dimensional approach to establish the shape as a sphere. This can be accomplished by obtaining a suprasternal notch echo for the left atrial Y dimension and a precordial echo for the Z dimension. Beware of the patient with a pectus excavatum, for this patient almost invariably will have an

unusually shaped left atrium. Usually it will be flattened in such a manner that the Y axis will be large with respect to the Z axis.

3. Always evaluate the right and left ventricular wall thickness and left ventricular wall and septal excursion.

4. Even though the mitral and tricuspid valves may be demonstrated without an obvious septum intervening, the septum may exist and may be totally intact (Fig. 4-5). Don't overdiagnose!

5. The left atrium can expand rapidly in an infant with decreasing pulmonary vascular resistance. Follow the suspect patients frequently.

6. When evaluating chamber sizes, the growth factor for left atrial and left ventricular dimension must be taken into account. With this in mind, serial determinations of left atrial size are meaningful.

Fig. 4-5. — No ventricular septal defect was found in this patient. This is a study of a normal child and demonstrates the fallibility of attempting to sight a "hole" in the septum where one can see the tricuspid valve anteriorly and the mitral valve posteriorly without a clear septum between. This sign may or may not be evidence for a ventricular septal defect. In this case it was not.

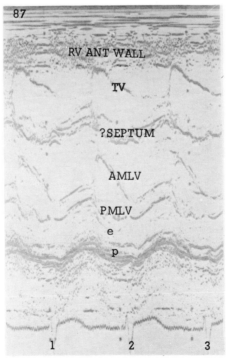

4.4. Single Ventricle

Pertinent literature references: 23, 24.

The echocardiographic diagnosis of single ventricle depends on demonstration of absence of a structure, the interventricular septum. Chesler and co-workers[23, 24] have stressed the abnormal motion of the anterior leaflet of the mitral valve. In the normal, the leaflet travel is restricted by the septum. In single ventricle, the anterior range of motion is increased.

Proving the absence of the structure always is more difficult than demonstrating structural abnormality or presence. Thus, even greater care must be used in arriving at this conclusion. Tricuspid and mitral valves should be recorded simultaneously to show absence of the septum. The anterior aortic wall should show no continuity to a septal-like structure. Both semilunar valves should be demonstrated.

Secondary features may aid in diagnosis. The great arteries in this condition may be transposed in either an "l" or a "d" location. The anterior right ventricular wall usually is thicker than normal. The atrioventricular valves may be unusual and frequently may have the configuration of the endocardial cushion defect. Occasionally, only one "common" atrioventricular valve is present.

Our Experience with This Lesion:

Most patients referred to us with this diagnosis have had a septum identified by echocardiography. Only a few patients with true single ventricle have been studied.

This is a complex group of patients who frequently have numerous defects, and thus the single ventricle is only part of a complex malformation. Transposition of an infundibular chamber is not uncommon, and a wall of this chamber may masquerade as part of the septum. Very large, high ventricular septal defects can act as and appear to be single ventricles, but usually a septum is found toward the apex or high near the aorta. If a septum is present, the diagnosis of single ventricle can be excluded. However, in some children and adults, the septum may not be found easily. In these individuals, one of the best techniques is to determine if any structure is continuous with the aorta. Abnormal papillary muscle structures at the apex may have the appearance of septal tissue; however, their chordal continuity with an atrioventricular valve sometimes can be used to differentiate them. These continuities demonstrate the necessity to scan or "sweep" the transducer and continuously record while doing this maneuver.

Points of Caution:

1. The diagnosis of single ventricle carries a very unfavorable prognosis. This fact puts the burden of proof on the echocardiographer to be correct.

2. In conditions such as mesoversion, L-transposition and dextrocardia, the septum is in a very abnormal location and alignment with respect to the normal. Diagnosis of absence of the septum is particularly likely to be made incorrectly in these instances, since the septum often is in a plane parallel to incident sound energy and produces no echoes that return toward the transducer.

3. The right ventricular cavity is small in the usual plane of examination, and if anterior resolution is limited, the anterior right ventricular wall, right ventricular cavity and septum may appear as a single structure echocardiographically, which could lead to a misdiagnosis of single ventricle. This can be avoided by use of high-frequency transducers, good technique and very careful examination. The anterior right ventricular wall rarely is more than a centimeter thick, and even a half centimeter is relatively uncommon. Any anterior right ventricular wall complex of greater than a centimeter should be scrutinized.

4. Septal identification in the patient with an endocardial cushion defect can be a problem, for the atrioventricular valves seem to pass through the septum. Careful superior and apical scanning usually will confirm the presence of a septum in these individuals.

5. Patients with hypoplastic right and left heart may seem to have a single ventricle. Anatomically, this is not true even though functionally it may be the case. The possibility of a hypoplastic right or left ventricle should be excluded to the maximal extent possible.

4.5. Endocardial Cushion Defect

Pertinent literature references: 37, 54, 88, 145, 176, 235.

Endocardial cushion defect is a generic term that includes all cardiac lesions created by the lack of fusion of the embryonic endocardial cushions. The spectrum of disease within the group is great and varies from the child with a small mitral cleft and a low atrial septal defect (ostium primum defect) to one with a total lack of endocardial cushion fusion. The total lack of fusion creates an atrial and ventricular septal defect and defects in the mitral and tricuspid valves. With respect to the valve leaflets, the cleft forms one end of the spectrum and a single primitive atrioventricular valve forms the other end. Papillary attachments usually are abnormal and the spectrum of attachment is quite variable. Almost every intermediate state is possible. Accordingly, the echocardiogram would not be expected to be similar in each variant.

Reports of Others:

Several reports have supplied the available echocardiographic information regarding the endocardial cushion defect. Gramiak and

Nanda[88] documented the echocardiograms of 5 adult patients in whom the outflow tract of the left ventricle was quite narrow. This finding is consistent with the "gooseneck deformity" seen on angiography. Williams and Rudd[235] found that the mitral valve excursion was not recorded best in the usual location as defined by interventricular landmarks. Additionally, they noted that mitral valve echoes, in cases in which there are dense attachments from the mitral leaflet to the crest of the interventricular septum, could be traced to the anterior border of the left ventricular outflow tract. They called this Type I anatomy. This finding, in part, confirms Gramiak and Nanda's conclusion in adult patients. One figure in Williams and Rudd's publication showed that the mitral valve forms the anterior border of the aortic root. This finding was said to be present in 6 of 7 patients studied with the strip chart recorder. In 14 of 28 patients, the anterior leaflet of the mitral valve could be traced superiorly to a typical-appearing mitral valve ring.

Patients with atrioventricular canal can demonstrate an unusual atrioventricular valve pattern. In systole, the mitral and tricuspid leaflets appear almost joined at about the level of the aortic root. In diastole, the mitral valve moves posteriorly whereas the tricuspid valve moves anteriorly. The mitral valve has a damped motion with short over-all excursion of less than 1 cm. The ventricular septum is absent between the leaflets.

Seven of 16 patients with complete atrioventricular canal showed an unusual pattern of atrioventricular motion that Williams and Rudd called Type II, in which a single atrioventricular valve leaflet was demonstrated in a posterior position in the left ventricle during systole and moved to a markedly anterior position in the right ventricle with the onset of diastole.

Williams and Rudd attributed the "gooseneck deformity" to the fact that the anterior mitral valve moved parallel rather than perpendicular to the septum. This raised the floor of the left ventricular outflow tract during diastole.

Eshaghpour et al.[54] reported multiple mitral echoes in late diastole and early systole. They also noted a rapid slope and large excursion of the mitral valve and large "V waves" in the posterior left atrial wall.

Pieroni and co-workers[176] reported four echocardiographic patterns of the mitral valve in endocardial cushion defect:

1. Exaggerated anterior mitral leaflet excursion traversing the interventricular septum.

2. Giant anterior mitral motion associated with reduced excursion of the tricuspid leaflet. The reverse pattern was less common but was

recorded also. They indicate that the predominant pattern depends on whether the common leaflet has a larger mitral or tricuspid component.

3. Double contour of the mitral valve in diastole was visualized and thought to represent the cleft portions of the valve.

4. Prolonged approximation of the anterior mitral valve to the interventricular septum in diastole. This unusual characteristic was thought to represent the anterior displacement of the cleft mitral valve.

Our Experience with This Lesion:

We have observed the expected echocardiographic variability in patients with this cardiac condition. Patients with ostium primum defects have demonstrated paradoxical septal motion and enlarged right ventricles.

In some patients, the mitral valve seems normal but in others the mitral valve motion is somewhat restrained in amplitude. In still others, the atrioventricular valve motion is greatly increased. The plane of the mitral valve is clearly different from normal, for the D–E slope can be recorded but the E–F slope is difficult to record, irrespective of transducer location. This finding may correspond to the comment of Eshaghpour et al.[54] This facet was shown, but not commented on, by Williams and Rudd in Figure 1 of their publication.[235]

One important finding in our patients has been the passage of the atrioventricular valve through the ventricular septum (Fig. 4-6). This is relatively characteristic of endocardial cushion defects and we have not visualized this in other lesions. The feature is recorded best near the aortic root. Occasionally we have observed Type I motion of Williams and Rudd, but, on finding this, we were able to demonstrate that changing the transducer angulation showed that the attachment is principally to the septum and not to the aortic root. Our finding is in general, but not in specific, accord with Williams and Rudd's comments. However, it is in accord with known anatomy. Type II of Williams and Rudd seems to be relatively common in the complete endocardial cushion defect.

In patients with the complete form of the lesion, the posterior left ventricular wall is difficult to align with the atrioventricular valve. Williams and Rudd's photographs also demonstrate this feature. This misalignment is due to the fact that the posterior left ventricular wall is not deep to the mitral valve. The mitral valve plane has been shifted. The right ventricular anterior wall frequently is thickened and the septum is difficult to follow from the apex to the aorta because of the large ventricular septal defect.

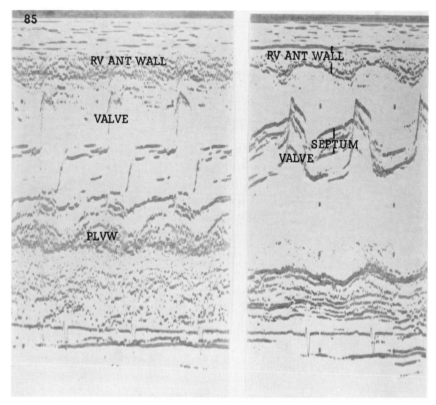

Fig. 4-6.—An endocardial cushion defect. Endocardial cushion defects come in a variety of types. This figure demonstrates two features of the endocardial cushion defect. In the left-hand panel is a very unusual valve that has a systolic position in the middle of the ventricle. Both valve portions move away from center during diastole. For an endocardial cushion defect, the one unusual feature of this example is the fact that the posterior left ventricular wall can be seen. Frequently, the wall cannot be visualized because the valve is displaced superiorly. The right-hand panel demonstrates the leaflet passing through the septum. This is a characteristic feature of the endocardial cushion defect. It is not clear which leaflet has this motion. Structure identification lines do not suggest measurement planes.

We have found only a few patients precisely like those described by Gramiak and Nanda.[88] However, the spectrum of the disease is so large that many more children with endocardial cushion defects will have to be studied before complete classifications can be developed.

Points of Caution:

1. The lesion is so anatomically variable that it is predictable that

a very wide spectrum of abnormal findings will be encountered by the echocardiographer.

2. The very wide mitral excursion that occurs in patients with mitral insufficiency of the nonendocardial cushion variety can be confused with the very wide excursion of the atrioventricular valve in the endocardial cushion defect. Since the left ventricular wall will be dilated with mitral insufficiency, the anterior left ventricular wall might be rotated even more anteriorly in that condition. These findings could simulate the appearance of an endocardial cushion defect.

3. We have observed some patients with endocardial cushion defects, usually those with primum defects, who have had echocardiographically normal-appearing atrioventricular valves.

4. Too little information is available, and the lesion is too variable, to be absolutely certain of the type of endocardial cushion defect from echocardiography. Two-dimensional echocardiography probably will be a superior tool in this lesion.

4.6. Total Anomalous Pulmonary Venous Return

Pertinent literature references: 79, 224.

Total anomalous pulmonary venous return is a severe form of right ventricular volume overload. One abstract[79] and one short publication[224] deal with this lesion. In the abstract, the authors suggest that 2 neonates with total anomalous pulmonary venous return had very small left atria with a total dimension of only 2 mm. Also, they reported excessive movement of the tricuspid valve and Type A paradoxical septal motion. These findings were thought to be diagnostic for echocardiography. Tajik et al.[224] reported an echocardiogram on a single patient with total anomalous pulmonary venous drainage. Their patient had paradoxical septal motion. They did not comment on the size of the left atrium.

Our Experience with This Lesion:

We have studied two patients with this defect. Left atrial size was normal in each. An additional chamber was visualized posterior to the left atrium.

Glaser and co-workers[79] have never published their findings in other than abstract form. Review of pathologic specimens shows that the left atrium is approximately normal in size and therefore would not have a dimension of 2 mm. Glaser et al. do not indicate the size of their children. If they were extremely small, perhaps smaller than 1000 gm, the 2-mm left atrium might be normal.

The reliability with which lesion can be diagnosed by echocardiography remains to be seen. It seems clear that not enough information concerning this lesion is available.

4.7. Valvular Aortic Stenosis

Pertinent literature references: 24, 90, 113, 165, 238, 239.

Valvular aortic stenosis is a highly variable lesion. The stenotic valve may have one to three cusps with variable degrees of adhesion. In children, the valve rarely is calcified. The configuration frequently is a dome that moves up and tenses with each systole and is retracted by cardiac relaxation in early diastole.

The motion of the aortic valve leaflet is relatively easy to record in normal children and in children with aortic stenosis. It is important to recognize that the space between the recorded leaflets of the aortic valve does not necessarily indicate the orifice size. In the normal, the systolic separation is only slightly dependent on where the beam transects the leaflet. However, if the valve leaflets are adhered and domed, transection of the lower portion of the leaflet by the beam would show the leaflets near or against the aortic wall. On the other hand, transection higher would show that the intercusp space was less (Fig. 7-10, A). With single crystal echocardiography it is virtually impossible to know precisely the level of beam transection of the aortic valve and therefore it is difficult to determine orifice size.

During diastole, normally closed aortic valves are shown by a single line, usually located in about mid-aortic lumen. Duplicated lines in diastole are rare but occur in the normal. When multiple diastolic lines are present, the aortic valve usually is abnormal.[238]

Normal aortic valves vibrate during systole. The significance of the frequency and amplitude of vibration is not entirely clear. Stenotic valves also vibrate and therefore this is not a differentiating feature.

Many children with aortic stenosis have bicuspid aortic valves. It has been suggested that these bicuspid valves may be diagnosed by demonstrating that the diastolic closure line is eccentrically placed in the lumen of the aorta.[165] This is based on the fact that, in most instances, one cusp or the other will predominate in size, and thus the orifice will be eccentrically located. Two potential problems with this concept are obvious.

1. The angle at which the beam passes through the aorta and the closed leaflets may vary from patient to patient and from transducer position to transducer position. This could give the erroneous appearance of one small and one large cusp.

2. Stenotic tricuspid semilunar valves usually are dissimilar in size. One cusp may be quite large and the remaining two may be

small or at least different in size. This could give the same echo representation as one large and one small bicuspid semilunar valve.

Calcification of the abnormal aortic valve is very rare in children. This lack of calcium causes the leaflet's motion to appear more normal. In the adult, calcification of the aortic valve produces a distinctive picture on the echocardiogram that consists of little leaflet separation[56] and multiple bright diastolic[90] leaflet echoes. Since the purpose of this book is to discuss the lesions that occur in children, we will not dwell on this particular aspect.

The secondary characteristics of aortic stenosis are of considerable echocardiographic importance. If the stenosis is of significance, patients usually have a thickened left ventricular posterior wall and septum[4] (Fig. 4-7). In the absence of congestive heart failure, the left

Fig. 4-7.—Severe left ventricular hypertrophy in a patient with aortic stenosis. This echocardiogram was obtained from a 2-month-old child with coarctation and aortic valvular stenosis. The cavity is small. Concentric hypertrophy is obvious. This child has very high end diastolic pressures. A prolonged A–C interval is present.

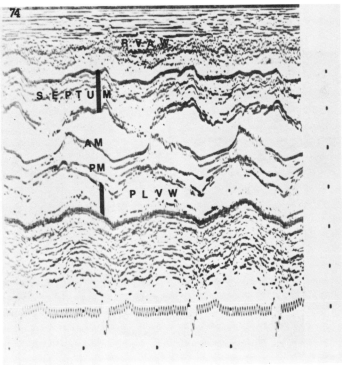

atrial dimension usually will be approximately normal. The aorta frequently is increased in dimension because of poststenotic dilatation.

Our Experience with This Lesion:

We have had the opportunity to perform echocardiograms on many children with congenital valvular aortic stenosis. Our results have been variable. Patients with mild aortic stenosis frequently have normal echocardiograms. Some have multiple diastolic lines (Fig. 4-8) and a few show minimal thickening of the left ventricular posterior wall and septum. The thickening usually is concentric and therefore the left ventricular wall and septum usually show approximately equal (symmetric) thickness as compared to asymmetric septal hypertrophy, in which the thickening of the septum is not matched by that of the left ventricular posterior wall.

Patients with moderately severe aortic stenosis usually have multiple diastolic lines, and the diastolic lines may be either eccentric or normally placed in the aortic lumen. The box-like configuration of the open aortic valve usually is preserved. Frequently it is extremely difficult to echo the top of the dome, probably because the top of the

Fig. 4-8.—Mild aortic stenosis in a 1-year-old boy. This picture demonstrates an abnormal aortic valve. Multiple eccentric diastolic lines are most obvious in beats 6 and 7. A central line during systole is visible in beats 1, 3, 4, 7 and possibly 6. Note that the cusp separation appears to be normal. The child had a systolic gradient of about 20 mm Hg.

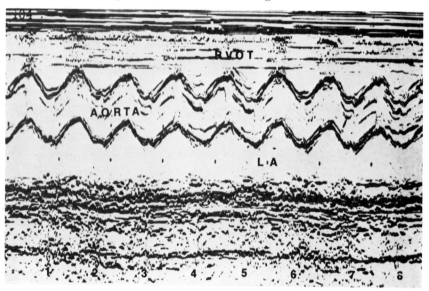

dome is relatively small by comparison with the walls of the dome. If we could find this point, the intercusp distance might be decreased, but usually we do not find the decreased intercusp distance.

Severe aortic stenosis almost always is detectable by echocardiography. The left ventricular posterior wall and septum usually are quite hypertrophied. The aortic valve separation may be small or may appear normal. The leaflets may appear thickened. However, the latter is a very subjective evaluation and is heavily dependent on the resolution of the equipment. The aorta usually is dilated.

We have investigated the eccentricity of the diastolic closure line in normal healthy children. We find that many of these children have an eccentric diastolic line. The location of the diastolic line of the aortic valve does not seem to predict the presence of or exclude bicuspid aortic valves.

The presence or absence of multiple diastolic lines frequently is a function of technique. It is possible to record single diastolic lines at one transducer angle and multiple lines at another angle (Fig. 4-9).

A thin third systolic line commonly is seen bisecting the aorta when the anterior and posterior leaflets are open. This has been considered to be the third cusp, which is not perpendicular to the sonar beam. However, unless this is the effect of excessive beam width, it is difficult to understand why this third cusp remains in the center of the aorta rather than moving toward the portion of the wall that is also parallel to the echo beam. We know of no validating evidence that would indicate that the third leaflet is truly the source of this line. It could even represent a phantom image of one of the other leaflets or the anterior aortic wall. This center line usually is fainter than the other leaflets and less well defined. The center line has also been seen in one of our patients with a unicuspid valve, and in this case (Fig. 4-10) it may have represented just another part of the aortic valve, which was to the side of the beam and not truly a leaflet. This explanation would be tenable in this particular instance, since the valve was domed and fixed and most portions did remain near the center of the aorta during systole. The same patient demonstrated the boxlike opening configuration. This is not surprising, for it merely represented the doming effect of the unicuspid valve.

A final maneuver that is helpful occasionally is cephalad angulation of the transducer beam in order to view the ascending aorta. In this manner, poststenotic dilatation of the aorta occasionally can be seen in valvular aortic stenosis.

Points of Caution:

1. Excellent recorder and instrument resolution are important

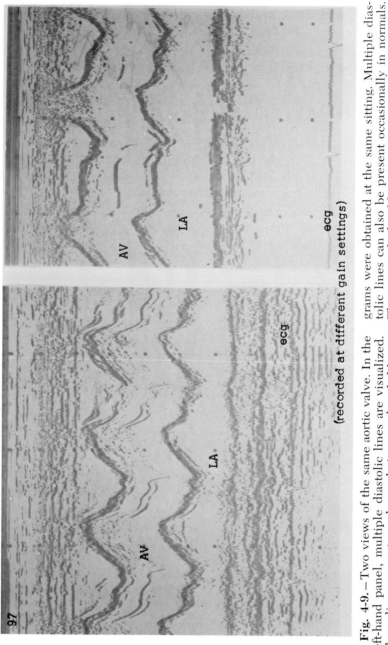

Fig. 4-9.—Two views of the same aortic valve. In the left-hand panel, multiple diastolic lines are visualized. These lines are not nearly as obvious, and probably are not present in the right-hand panel. Both echocardiograms were obtained at the same sitting. Multiple diastolic lines can also be present occasionally in normals. This patient had mild aortic stenosis.

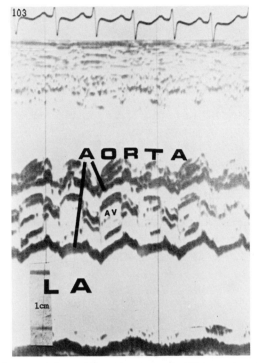

Fig. 4-10.—Severe unicuspid aortic stenosis. This patient had a distorted aortic valve, and multiple diastolic lines are seen. There is a third line between the anterior and posterior aortic valve cusps. He had a unicuspid valve at operation. The origin of the center line is not certain.

when studying the aortic valve. Poor resolution, especially by Polaroid, can make normal leaflets appear thickened. Estimating leaflet thickness is difficult even with excellent equipment.

2. Even the tightest aortic stenosis can produce the normal box-like configuration because of the doming effect of the lower portion of the valve.

3. A strip chart recorder is almost essential for studying the small child because a large number of complexes must be evaluated carefully. It is difficult to capture an adequate number on Polaroid prints.

4. Evaluation of the effects of aortic stenosis on the left ventricular posterior wall and septum is as important as observation of the valve itself.

5. The possibility of aortic stenosis cannot be ruled out because the echocardiogram seems normal.

6. Eccentric diastolic aortic valve lines occur frequently in normal healthy children.

7. Multiple diastolic lines occur occasionally in normals.

4.8. Aortic Insufficiency

Pertinent literature references: 33, 56, 65, 69, 90, 113, 117, 132, 190, 237.

Congenital and/or acquired aortic insufficiency present similar echocardiographic features. Little, if any, information can be gained by directly viewing the aortic valve, although dilatation of the aortic root may occur in some cases of aortic insufficiency. Depending on the severity of insufficiency and the compliance of the left ventricle, varying dilatation of the left ventricle may occur. It has been reported that approximately one-third of the patients with chronic aortic insufficiency have vibration of the anterior mitral valve leaflet along its E – F slope.[237] Fortuin and Craige[69] have shown that in patients with increased left ventricular end diastolic pressure, the anterior mitral valve drifts more toward a position of closure during diastole. Thus, during the "passive filling" phase, the valve is in a partially closed position. A murmur results from blood flowing across the partially closed valve. Further, as volume and pressure increase in the left ventricle, the valve still is partially closed and atrial contraction causes still another murmur. The aortic insufficiency murmur and the presystolic murmur combine to create the Austin Flint murmur.

An elegant study on left ventricular function in aortic insufficiency was done by Danford et al.[33] In this study, they calculated left ventricular output by Fortuin's formula[71] and subtracted mitral valve flow, which they determined by the formula

$$Q = AVT$$

where A = mitral valve cross-sectional area (assumed to be 5 cm^2 in the adult), V = blood velocity across the mitral valve, which equals the anterior mitral valve opening velocity in cm/sec, and T = the duration of flow across the mitral valve in seconds.

The assumptions necessary for this include:

1. Laminar flow.

2. Opening mitral valve velocity represents linear velocity.

3. Leaflets lack inertia.

4. Flow is constant throughout ventricular filling.

Using these assumptions, Kingsley[132] found that stroke volume and cardiac output varied no more than 15% from outputs determined from dye curves in 500 patients. The implications from this paper are important in that this may represent a noninvasive method of calculating regurgitant volume, which is a difficult parameter to calculate by invasive means at present.

Our Experience with This Lesion:

We have seen anterior mitral valve leaflet vibration only occasionally. Two types were noted. The first was a high-frequency, high-amplitude vibration (Fig. 4-11). The second was a low-frequency, moderate-amplitude type (Fig. 4-12). Left ventricular dilatation usu-

Fig. 4-11.—Fine vibration in severe aortic insufficiency. The patient is a 16-year-old girl with very severe rheumatic aortic insufficiency. Note the fine high-frequency vibration of the anterior mitral valve (multiple echoes) and the large left ventricular internal dimension. High-frequency mitral valve vibration, in our experience, is about as common as low-frequency vibration in patients with aortic insufficiency.

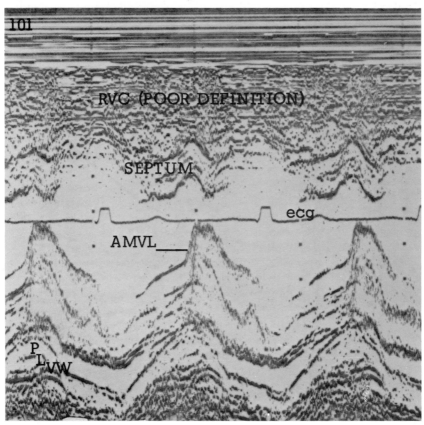

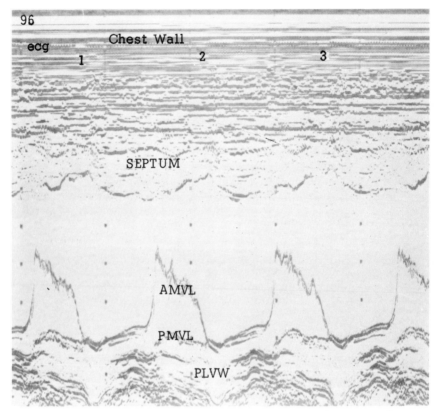

Fig. 4-12. — Aortic insufficiency in a 13-year-old boy. This echocardiogram shows an example of low-frequency vibration of the mitral valve. This was taken from a boy who had less severe aortic insufficiency than was shown in Figure 4-11. Severity and frequency of vibration do not seem to be correlated in aortic insufficiency.

ally has been present and sometimes is very marked. In 2 patients with chronic aortic insufficiency, presumably rheumatic, without mitral insufficiency, we have observed decreased Vcf, which we believe is on a basis of congestive heart failure. These patients had increased left ventricular end diastolic pressure at cardiac catheterization. As more experience is gained with Vcf, it may be a useful parameter to follow. Danford's approach has yet to be applied to the pediatric patient.

Points of Caution:
1. Acquired conditions frequently are associated with aortic insuf-

ficiency. The primary disease may cause left ventricular dilatation (for example, rheumatic carditis).

2. Some vibration or fluttering of the anterior mitral valve leaflet can be seen in normals and in atrial fibrillation, and it is not seen in all patients with aortic insufficiency.

3. Aortic insufficiency varies in clinical and hemodynamic expression. So will its echo expression.

4. This is another example of echocardiographic manifestations of a specific lesion being reflected indirectly by the mitral valve and left ventricle. Such secondary signs point out the importance of a careful, thorough, echocardiographic examination of each patient.

5. Subacute bacterial endocarditis can cause aortic insufficiency. Vegetations can be seen in some cases. Carefully examine the entire aortic valve for vegetations whenever subacute bacterial endocarditis is suspected.

6. Vibration is a relatively subjective finding. The extent to which it may be normal and above which it is abnormal is not easily quantitated. It can be masked by poor resolution recording.

4.9. Subaortic Stenosis

Pertinent literature references: 34, 145, 185, 227.

Subaortic stenosis occurs in two basic forms:

1. Discrete (membranous or fibromuscular tunnel).

2. Variable (idiopathic hypertrophic subaortic stenosis).

The variable form will be discussed as idiopathic hypertrophic subaortic stenosis. The discrete form is the subject of this section.

The membranous form usually is a thin diaphragm attached to the anterior mitral valve leaflet and the septum high in the outflow tract of the left ventricle. An orifice is present in the diaphragm and the jet of blood that passes through that orifice frequently strikes and eventually damages the aortic valve so as to make it incompetent.

Several investigators have studied this defect with echocardiography. Popp and co-workers[185] reported the results in 3 patients and demonstrated echocardiograms. One had a discrete membrane, one had a fibrous membrane with hypertrophied muscle bundles and the other had a fibromuscular tunnel. The echocardiogram for the patient with the simple diaphragm (Fig. 4-13) showed a high-intensity echo in the left ventricular outflow tract connected to the anterior mitral valve leaflet. This echo moved anteriorly with systole and posteriorly with diastole. The tracing for the patient with a fibrous membrane and hypertrophied muscle bundles,showed outflow tract narrowing with systole near the free edge of the anterior mitral valve

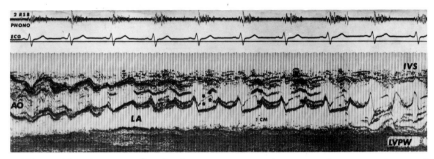

Fig. 4-13. – An example of subaortic stenosis. An unusual structure is noted that has an anterior motion during systole and is identified by four arrows. It is clearly in the outflow tract of the left ventricle and seems to disappear lower in the ventricle. This structure is thought to be the subaortic diaphragm. Phonocardiogram is also demonstrated. An unidentified dense echo is also noted in the left ventricular outflow tract. (Dr. Richard Popp kindly provided this photograph for use. Also, by the courtesy of *Circulation*.[185])

leaflet, but narrowing did not occur at the annulus. The echocardiogram of the patient with the tunnel showed a very narrow left ventricular outflow tract, which widened after surgery.

Davis and co-workers[34] reported results in 3 patients with discrete subaortic membranes. They found abnormal movement of the aortic valve leaflets, which consisted of partial premature closure shortly after the onset of ventricular systole. Following operation on 2 of these patients, the leaflets still showed premature closure, but the degree was less than preoperatively. In contrast to Popp and co-workers,[185] they observed unusual but inconsistent findings in the left ventricular outflow tract.

Our Experience with This Lesion:

We attempted to but have not observed the signs suggested by Popp *et al.* and Davis *et al.* in 3 patients with diaphragms. In two instances, these diaphragms caused minor gradients and in a third the gradient was significant. Our patients had thick left ventricular walls as their only abnormal finding. The aortic valve looked approximately normal.

On occasion, in other patients, we have seen the unusual early wide opening of the aortic valve followed by abrupt near closure in the first half of systole. The reason for this is not clear. How pathognomonic the aortic valve signs remain for subaortic stenosis is yet to be proved.

Points of Caution:

1. From the results of Popp and co-workers, it is clear that the diaphragm can be found, but this is neither easy nor uniformly possible.

2. The aortic valve sign can be seen in other lesions. Specifically, we have seen it most commonly in patients with ventricular septal defects and left-to-right shunts. We also observed that the posterior semilunar valve in a patient with transposition, pulmonary hypertension and ventricular septal defect had a configuration almost precisely like that reported by Davis *et al.* for subaortic diaphragms.

3. Patients with hypoplastic left heart may have narrow outflow tracts of the left ventricle that have some similarity to the fibromuscular tunnel. However, in hypoplastic left heart, the entire ventricle is hypoplastic, and not just the outflow tract.

4.10. Idiopathic Hypertrophic Subaortic Stenosis (IHSS) and Asymmetric Septal Hypertrophy

Pertinent literature references: 2, 3, 13, 17, 29, 34, 93, 101, 102, 140, 161, 189, 191, 204, 205, 228.

Numerous publications regarding echocardiographic diagnosis of asymmetric septal hypertrophy have appeared. A comprehensive evaluation of the problem was presented by Henry and co-workers.[101] They evaluated the ratio of septal to left ventricular posterior wall thickness in normals, patients with fixed left ventricular outflow obstruction and in patients with IHSS. Normals had approximately equal thickness of the septum and left ventricular posterior wall. Patients with IHSS, about half of whom had no gradient at rest, had a ratio of septal to left ventricular posterior wall thickness of greater than 1.3:1 (Fig. 4-14). On the basis of these data, they classified individuals with a septum to left ventricular posterior wall thickness ratio of greater than 1.3:1 as having asymmetric septal hypertrophy. Brown and co-workers pointed out that the ratio must take into account the possibility of right ventricular hypertrophy, for the septum may also thicken as part of the hypertrophy of the right heart.[17, 85]

IHSS is a condition characterized by variable subaortic obstruction of the outflow from the left ventricle. Genetically, the condition is a dominant with nearly complete penetrance if all forms of the disease are taken into account.[101] The most complete form is characterized by thickened ventricular septum and obstruction to left ventricular outflow.[3, 101, 161, 191, 204] The anterior mitral valve leaflet and the septum contribute to the obstruction.[102] The "nonobstructive" form, possibly the precursor of this complete form, is asymmetric septal hypertrophy, which usually does not produce a measurable obstruction to left ventricular outflow. However, patients with asymmetric septal hypertrophy may develop a gradient under certain conditions and may exhibit characteristic echocardiographic findings of IHSS.

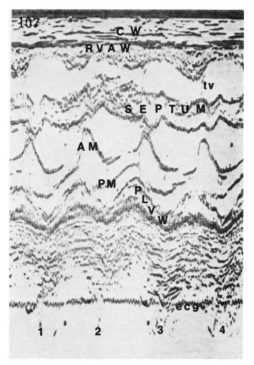

Fig. 4-14.—This is an example of a child whose mother has asymmetric septal hypertrophy. Unlike some infants whose septal hypertrophy disappears with time, this child's did not. Note that the septum is considerably thicker than the posterior left ventricular wall at the level of the anterior and posterior leaflets of the mitral valve *(AM, PM)*. The septum is not thick as the result of right ventricular hypertrophy, for the right ventricular anterior wall *(RVAW)* is not abnormally thickened. A portion of the tricuspid value *(tv)* is shown.

When a patient with asymmetric septal hypertrophy has a pressure gradient, systolic anterior motion (SAM) of the mitral valve frequently can be identified by echocardiography.[101, 102, 204] The most characteristic location of SAM is at the edge of the mitral valve leaflet [204] at approximately the same level as the posterior mitral valve leaflet. If the echo beam is directed more superiorly than the point at which the posterior mitral valve leaflet is sighted, mitral annulus is encountered. This structure normally moves anteriorly during systole. Thus, care must be used in selecting the portion of the anterior mitral valve leaflet for study. In individuals with IHSS, the anterior mitral valve leaflet approaches the septum and may appear to nearly, or even completely, occlude the left ventricular outflow tract[102] (Fig. 4-15). However, total occlusion is more apparent than real, for the single transducer echocardiogram cannot record all of the surfaces of the anterior mitral valve leaflet simultaneously. Henry and co-workers[102] developed an obstruction index that takes into account the duration

Fig. 4-15. — This is an example of IHSS (idiopathic hypertrophic subaortic stenosis). During systole, the anterior leaflet of the mitral valve shows systolic anterior motion (SAM). The septum and posterior left ventricular wall are quite thickened. This patient has a normal septal to posterior wall ratio. One centimeter markers are shown at the right. The endocardial surface (E) is marked. A carotid tracing and phonocardiogram are demonstrated. (We are indebted to Dr. Bertron Groves for this photograph.)

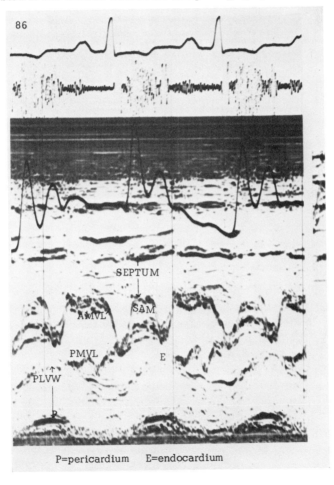

P=pericardium   E=endocardium

of the SAM and the separation of the anterior mitral leaflet and the septum. This index correlates with the pressure gradient measured at cardiac catheterization. The obstruction index is equal to duration of outflow narrowing /mean septal-anterior mitral valve leaflet distance. The gradient is equal to $(1.8) \times$ (obstruction index) -35.

Many patients with significant obstruction eject much of their cardiac output during early systole. In these patients, premature systolic closure of the aortic valve may be seen as obstruction increases.

Our Experience with This Lesion:

IHSS is not common in children, but its precursor, asymmetric septal hypertrophy, is relatively common in families in which a member has IHSS or asymmetric septal hypertrophy. Demonstration of characteristic SAM of the anterior mitral valve leaflet is not particularly difficult when it is present. However, it is not always present in patients with transitional forms. Demonstration may require provocative testing with a drug such as amyl nitrite.

Asymmetric septal hypertrophy is a diagnosis that must be made with extreme caution in children. If it is strictly defined as a ratio of septum to left ventricular posterior wall thickness of greater than 1.3:1, we have demonstrated it in the following conditions: ventricular septal defect, patent ductus arteriosus, coarctation of the aorta, tetralogy of Fallot, transposition and pulmonic stenosis. Most of these patients also had right ventricular hypertrophy. Even more important, we have seen the abnormal ratio in normal, healthy neonates with no familial history (Fig. 4-16). This type disappears with time. We are reluctant to make a diagnosis of asymmetric septal hypertrophy in the newborn or in any child who has associated right ventricular hypertrophy.

We concur with Henry *et al.*'s finding that if a proband with true IHSS is found, about half of the siblings and one of the parents will exhibit asymmetric septal hypertrophy or IHSS. As septal hypertrophy may be progressive, children with borderline septal to posterior wall ratios as well as unaffected siblings should be scheduled for repeated examinations at appropriate intervals. Finally, obstructive IHSS may be present with a normal septal to posterior wall thickness ratio.

Points of Caution:

1. The systolic anterior motion must arise from the anterior mitral valve leaflet. At times, it is possible to see the mitral annulus and both leaflets of the mitral valve simultaneously. This superimposition of structures may falsely simulate systolic anterior motion of IHSS.

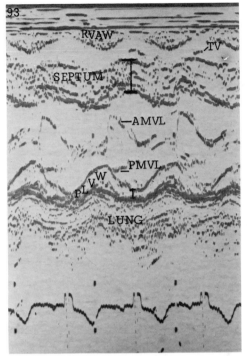

Fig. 4-16. — An example of apparent asymmetric septal hypertrophy in a normal neonate. The echocardiogram showed a thick septum with respect to the thickness of the left ventricular posterior wall. We obtained normal measurements from the parents and grandmother. This pattern persisted for approximately 2 months, and then the child demonstrated loss of septal thickening. Six months later his ratio was 0.9:1.

2. Do not diagnose asymmetric septal hypertrophy if right ventricular hypertrophy is present. Right ventricular hypertrophy can include septal hypertrophy.[17] Therefore, the right ventricular anterior wall must be visualized and measured.

3. Be cautious of a tricuspid leaflet that "appears" to be part of the ventricular septum, thus making the septum appear abnormally thick (Fig. 4-17).

4. Look for SAM only when the mitral valve leaflets are recorded simultaneously.

5. Beware of the diagnosis of asymmetric septal hypertrophy in the newborn, even if the anterior right ventricular wall is thin. Also, be wary of the diagnosis of asymmetric septal hypertrophy when the septum is of normal thickness.

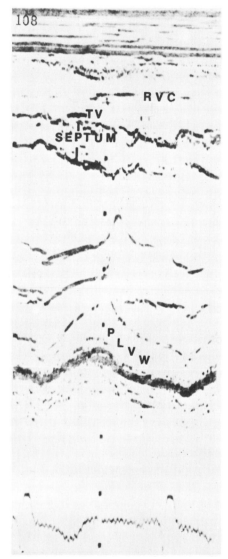

Fig. 4-17. – Possible confusion of tricuspid valve and septum. A small portion of the tricuspid valve can be seen above the septum. Misidentification of the valve could lead one to misdiagnose a falsely thickened septum.

6. Provocative testing may be necessary to elicit systolic anterior motion of the anterior mitral valve leaflet.

7. Since the diagnosis of asymmetric septal hypertrophy is dependent on the ratio of the left ventricular posterior wall and the sep-

tum, very clearly defined structures are required for accurate measurement.

8. Pseudosystolic anterior motion of the anterior mitral valve leaflet may occur in patients who have atrial septal defects and normal mitral valve function.

4.11. Aortic Root Dissection

Pertinent literature references: 56, 122, 160, 166, 245.

Aortic root dissection is an uncommon pediatric problem, although it can occur in patients with cystic medial necrosis, especially in males.[122]

Few reports of dissection are present in the literature [56, 160, 166, 245] but the findings in the patients reported are consistent. The first report by Millward et al.[160] showed that instead of the two parallel moving aortic walls, two anterior and two posterior parallel moving lines are recorded. The degree of separation of the intima from the outer wall depends on the amount and site of dissection.

Nanda et al.[166] state that the aortic root is dilated beyond normal and the affected wall is widened beyond normal limits.

Yuste et al.[245] performed echoes on a young man, preoperatively and postoperatively, and showed that the double anterior and posterior walls returned to normal after primary repair of the lesion.

In his text, Feigenbaum[56] states that the findings of aortic dissection are not constant.

Although Marfan's syndrome and cystic medial necrosis can also be associated with dissecting aneurysm of the pulmonary artery, no reports of this entity have reached the echo literature.

Our Experience with This Lesion:
We have no experience with this lesion at present.
Points of Caution:
1. The aortic walls frequently seem thick.
2. False positives are common.

4.12. Mitral Disease

Pertinent literature references: *Mitral Stenosis*
45, 46, 47, 48, 51, 56, 57, 96, 142, 143, 144, 168, 169, 201, 213.
Mitral Insufficiency
9, 56, 77, 116, 127, 157, 159, 203, 225, 227.

Mitral Stenosis:
Most of the early echocardiographic literature was devoted to acquired rheumatic mitral stenosis.

Edler[48] showed that patients with mitral stenosis had decreased E – F mitral valve slopes. The slope correlated inversely with the severity of the stenosis. Gustafson[96] correlated calculated mitral valve areas for patients with mitral stenosis who were in sinus rhythm and related the results to their E – F slopes. He found a positive correlation between the slope and the valve area (r = 0.62). After commissurotomy,[46, 51, 96, 234] the E – F slope increased. Thus, the E – F slope is useful as a predictor of stenosis or restenosis[56] (Fig. 4-18). However, a decreased mitral E – F slope can occur in conditions other than mitral stenosis. These include aortic stenosis and aortic

Fig. 4-18. – Example of moderate mitral stenosis. This example demonstrates anterior motion of the posterior mitral valve leaflet in diastole. The E – F slope of the anterior mitral valve leaflet is 48 mm/sec. Note that the patient has atrial fibrillation, accounting for varying diastolic times. Time lines are 1 second. Calibration markers are to the right of the photograph.

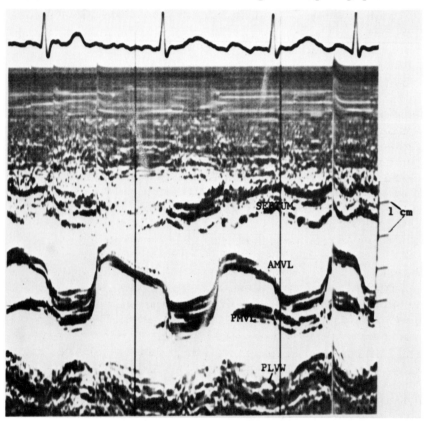

insufficiency with increased left ventricular end diastolic pressure, idiopathic hypertrophic subaortic stenosis, pulmonary hypertension and atrial septal defects. All are associated with a "pseudo mitral stenosis" pattern.

Duchak et al.[45] added the important observation that it is necessary to view the posterior mitral valve leaflet as well as the anterior mitral valve leaflet. Normally, these leaflets move apart. In true mitral stenosis, the leaflets are somewhat fused and move essentially in the same anterior direction in diastole. The posterior mitral leaflet appears to be tucked into the anterior mitral leaflet on the echocardiogram (Fig. 4-18).

Congenital mitral stenosis has been reported to have the same characteristics as the acquired form in one report.[142] In another,[213] the hypoplastic mitral valve did not open until atrial systole occurred because of the high left ventricular end diastolic pressure. In 7 cases of congenital mitral stenosis, Lundström[143] noted decreased mitral amplitude and decreased E–F velocity. These slopes and amplitudes improved after valvotomy. He did not show the posterior mitral valve leaflet in his figures.

Mitral Insufficiency:

Mitral insufficiency can result from many etiologies. According to some, the E–F anterior mitral valve slope is exaggerated in mitral insufficiency.[9, 46, 50, 119, 203] However, Feigenbaum states that any condition associated with increased mitral flow will increase the E–F slope. A Chinese publication[225] states that normal left atrial posterior wall motion is flat and fairly straight. A phenomenon was observed in mitral insufficiency consisting of a systolic "downward deflection" of the left atrial posterior wall. The depression was called "C-sink" and resulted from systolic distention of the left atrium by the mitral insufficiency. C-sink was found in 20.6% of normals, in 6.7% of patients with mitral stenosis, and in 87% of patients with mitral stenosis and insufficiency. To further separate conditions, they observed the time interval between the electrocardiographic R wave and the backward left atrial posterior wall motion (Rb interval) and found it to be longer in normals than in patients with mitral insufficiency. Bc amplitude is the depth of C-sink and represents the extent of backward movement of the left atrial posterior wall in systole. This is less pronounced in normals and in patients with mitral stenosis than in those with mitral insufficiency.

Johnson et al.[116] use a directional range-gated pulsed Doppler to detect mitral insufficiency. A harsh systolic jet is detected when the Doppler beam is directed into the left atrium in patients with mitral insufficiency. This qualitatively correlated well with mitral insufficiency found at catheterization. The technique allows localization of the origin of murmurs and may hold great future promise, especially if quantitation is possible.

Our Experience with These Lesions:

We have seen no patients with congenital mitral stenosis other than those with hypoplastic left heart. Acquired mitral insufficiency has been seen in numerous patients with myocarditis and myocardiopathies, including rheumatic. We have not been helped by the velocity or amplitude of the mitral valve. However, indirect evidence is very useful. Left ventricular posterior wall and septal excursion may increase markedly. The left atrial and ventricular cavities are dilated. Left atrial cavity size seems to closely mirror the extent of insufficiency. Aortic insufficiency can cause the same left ventricular findings. If the patient with aortic insufficiency develops congestive heart failure, the left atrium may dilate, but usually to a lesser degree than is caused by mitral insufficiency.

Congestive cardiomyopathy and mitral valve prolapse are specific forms of mitral insufficiency. These are discussed elsewhere.

Points of Caution:

1. When observing a patient for mitral stenosis, be sure to evaluate the posterior mitral valve leaflet, as decreased E–F anterior mitral valve leaflet slope can be found in many conditions.

2. Atrial myxomas can be confused with mitral stenosis if the thin normal anterior mitral valve leaflet is missed and only the rounded tumor edge is seen.

3. Unless there is mitral prolapse or congestive cardiomyopathy, mitral insufficiency is not a primary echo diagnosis. Other causes of left atrial and left ventricular volume overload should be sought clinically. Examples include ventricular septal defect, patent ductus arteriosus and aortic insufficiency.

4. Serial follow-up is more useful than a single examination. Mitral stenosis or insufficiency can be progressive.

4.13. Prolapse of the Mitral Valves

Pertinent literature references: 9, 36, 40, 56, 180.

Prolapsed mitral valve is a rather common condition in children and usually is associated with a midsystolic click and/or a late systolic murmur. The angiographic picture is one of prolapse of the posterior[40] and sometimes the anterior[36] mitral valve leaflets into the left atrium during the latter part of systole. Pathologically, these valve leaflets are redundant and often show myxomatous degeneration. This is an important lesion, for:

1. It is a type of mitral insufficiency that can be specifically defined by echocardiography, and

2. Some patients with this lesion are subject to serious arrhythmias.

Normal mitral valve leaflets exhibit a slow anterior motion during systole. This is demonstrated by single or multiple parallel lines. The parallel lines are due to the fact that the ultrasound beam subtends more than one surface of the mitral valve leaflets (Fig. 4-19). Thus, recording multiple mitral lines during systole does not indicate the presence of mitral insufficiency. Further, as the leaflets coapt only near their free edges, recordings above this area normally may show some systolic separation. Individuals with prolapse of the mitral valve usually have initially normal systolic motion of the leaflets, but in midsystole, the posterior mitral valve leaflet and occasionally the anterior mitral valve leaflet sag posteriorly into the left atrium. In a few patients, the prolapse begins early in systole.[180] At, or just prior to, the completion of systole, the leaflets assume an anterior motion and demonstrate normal diastolic motion.[40, 56] In some patients, both leaflets may show general "sagging" or "hammock-like" systolic motion profiles, with or without discrete late systolic prolapse.[180] Furthermore, multiple prolapsed segments may be seen

Fig. 4-19. — Multiple echoes from the mitral valve. The mitral valve is shown diagrammatically. The lowest beam would strike only the combined cusps and would produce a single echo. If the beam were aimed slightly higher, the mitral valves would be subtended in four points as marked. A still higher beam might catch only the tops and produce two echoes. Numbers refer to intersected sites at each level. The heavy, lowest line diagrammatically represents the valve annulus.

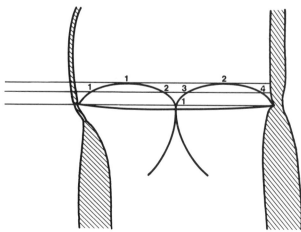

in patients who have multiple clicks. Both mitral leaflets must be recorded simultaneously to make the diagnosis of posterior prolapse. The best recordings usually are accomplished at or just below the level of juncture between the left atrium and the left ventricle (Fig. 4-20).

Although the diagnosis can be suspected clinically and proved by angiography, this lesion is particularly well suited to diagnosis by echocardiography.

If insufficiency is significant, the left atrium and left ventricle may be dilated.

Our Experience with This Lesion:

The frequency of prolapse is more common than we expected. Usually it is relatively easy to prove, but some individuals demonstrate the characteristic pattern of the leaflet motion only part of the time. For this reason, it is wise to listen to the patient just before attempting to perform the echocardiogram to be certain that the click and murmur are present at examination time. Provocation of the insufficiency by increasing systemic resistance may produce characteristic echocardiographic findings in individuals with mild forms of this condition. Likewise, amyl nitrite inhalation, which decreases end systolic volume by lowering systemic resistance, may accentuate the findings.

One frustrating feature of this condition is that, at times, the posterior leaflet and the posterior left atrial wall blend into a common line. When this happens, the echocardiographer cannot be certain of the diagnosis. Changing the patient's position may alter the anatomic relationship or circulation sufficiently to permit easier diagnosis.

Although we have seen this condition in the very young child, it seems more common after 3 years of age.

Points of Caution:

1. Do not confuse the posterior mitral valve leaflet with the left atrial wall.

2. Always record both leaflets simultaneously.

3. Some children have almost flat systolic motion of the mitral valve normally.

4. If the murmur and click are absent at the time of examination, have the patient squat or perform an isometric exercise.

5. If the syndrome seems to be present by physical examination but not present by echocardiography, even with provocative maneuvers, evaluate the tricuspid valve.

6. This condition is relatively common in patients with pectus excavatum, but obtaining a diagnostic study may be difficult because of the cardiac distortion introduced by the chest deformity.

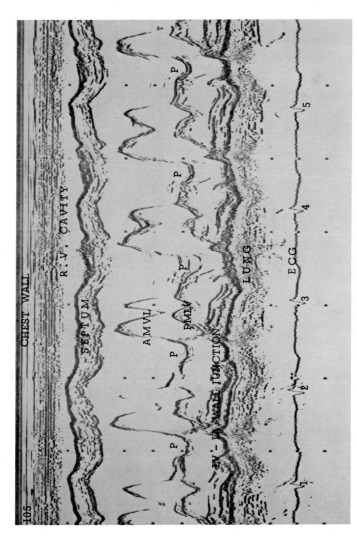

Fig. 4-20.—Multiple views of mitral valve prolapse in a 7-year-old girl with midsystolic click and murmur. This echocardiogram demonstrates a number of different views of prolapse in subsequent beats. In the first beat, the prolapse is obvious, but not nearly as remarkable as in beats 3 and 4. In those beats, multiple prolapse lines are noted. This echocardiogram was taken from the area of the left ventricular-left atrial junction, which is a proper place to look for prolapse. P = prolapse.

7. This motion abnormality should be searched for in preoperative and postoperative patients with atrial septal defects.

4.14. Flail Mitral Leaflet

Pertinent literature references: 44, 56, 215.

This is a rare lesion in children, although it may be seen occasionally after subacute bacterial endocarditis. In the adult, the abnormal posterior mitral leaflet moves posteriorly in systole and remains there until diastole begins.[44, 215] In prolapse, the posterior leaflet usually initially moves anteriorly during systole and then prolapses. The flail mitral leaflet overshoots anteriorly during early diastole and then remains flat.

If chordae of the anterior leaflet are severed, erratic fluttering occurs during diastole.[44] Feigenbaum[56] reports a notch on the tracing of the anterior mitral valve leaflet echo after the E point in this condition.

4.15. Cor Triatriatum

Pertinent literature references: 143, 163.

Cor triatriatum is considered to result from faulty development of the atrial septum or failure of normal incorporation of the embryologic common pulmonary vein into the left atrium. Anatomically, cor triatriatum has an accessory chamber that varies in size depending on:

1. The orifice of the diaphragm, which separates the pulmonary venous receiving chamber from the left atrium, or

2. The presence and location of an atrial septal defect.[163]

If there is no egress of pulmonary venous blood, the pulmonary venous collecting chamber will be dilated. If there is a route of egress, it will be decompressed and of normal or near normal size.

There is one echocardiographic report of a patient with cor triatriatum in the literature.[143] An echo 7 mm posterior to the mitral valve was noted to move with atrial events. The left atrium itself was not viewed, however, and the photographs are difficult to interpret. Further work is necessary to determine the usefulness of echo in cor triatriatum.

Our Experience with This Lesion:

Specifically, we have had none in uncorrected patients. We have echocardiographically examined a patient with a closed chamber that had an appendage, foramen ovale and received the pulmonary veins. Below this chamber was an atrioventricular canal. Our patient technically had a stenosing ring of the left atrium. As there was no egress of pulmonary venous drainage, the echo showed a large chamber posterior to the aorta. Mitral valve motion was seen below the chamber but no specific membrane could be found, although we knew it was present. Although this case does not represent true cor triatriatum, the echocardiographic appearance should be similar, especially if the chamber has no decompression.

Points of Caution:

1. There is insufficient information to echocardiographically diagnose this lesion at present. If it is suspected, angiography probably still is necessary to make this diagnosis.

2. As the lesion is variable in expression, so will be the echo findings.

3. Complete echocardiograms are necessary and must include full evaluation of the left atrium. Suprasternal notch echocardiography *may* show a diaphragm above the mitral valve. It did not in our patient.

4.16. Pulmonary Stenosis

Pertinent literature references: 89, 233.

The pulmonary valve was the last of the four cardiac valves evaluated echocardiographically, mainly because it is difficult to record and interpret. As indicated in Chapter 3, it is much more common to see two leaflets of the pulmonary valve in the neonate than in older children. Cusp separation has not been suggested as an echocardiographic criterion of pulmonary stenosis. It is predicted that the diagnosis of stenosis on this basis would be fraught with the same difficulties that have been mentioned for the aortic valve. Briefly, the stenotic semilunar valves frequently are domed. Therefore, the leaflets at the base of the dome appear to separate widely, but at the top of the dome they adhere. No reference point is available to determine the portion of the dome being viewed. This is unfortunate, for the orifice at the top of the dome may be quite small with respect to the separation of the walls of the dome.

Weyman *et al.*[233] indicated that it is possible to obtain information regarding stenosis by observing the posterior leaflet of the pulmonary valve. Gramiak *et al.*[89] reported that the normal posterior leaflet moves posteriorly with right atrial contraction. Movement occurs because the pressure and resistance in the normal pulmonary artery at end diastole is low. The inflow of blood created by atrial systole causes the pulmonary valve to be tensed or even opened before the right ventricle begins to contract. If the pressure difference between the right ventricle and the pulmonary artery is considerable, as in pulmonary stenosis, the presystolic, posterior bulge may become pronounced.[233] Normal posterior motion ranged from 0 to 7 mm. Motion in patients with gradients of 50–142 mm ranged from 8 to 13 mm. The leaflet did not return to the closed position prior to ventricular systole in patients with gradients greater than 65 mm Hg. Weyman *et al.* presented echocardiograms to demonstrate this feature. They indicated that the more severe the stenosis the greater the maximal presystolic posterior motion of the pulmonary valve. Their population included 14 patients with pulmonary stenosis, 18 normals and 65 patients with other cardiac diseases. To date, this is the only reported echocardiographic demonstration of pulmonary stenosis.

Our Experience with This Lesion:

We concur with Weyman *et al.*'s finding that the presystolic posterior motion of the posterior leaflet of the pulmonary valve can be accentuated in patients with pulmonary stenosis. However, we have also noted that this is not always present. Figure 4-21 demonstrates echocardiograms of the pulmonary valve in 4 patients with pulmonary stenosis, gradient 35–100 mm Hg. None has a very impressive presystolic posterior motion. Perhaps at higher gradients the bulge would be more noticeable, but a 100-mm gradient is a very significant pulmonary stenosis. Figure 4-22 demonstrates the pulmonary valve in another patient with pulmonary stenosis. This patient sometimes demonstrates the posterior motion and sometimes does not.

Feigenbaum concluded that the relative pressure in the two chambers produced the bulge. This is plausible. However, some valves are so stenotic and thick that this bulge might not occur. Thus, the actual histopathology of the valve probably is important in the creation of the presystolic posterior bulge.

An important secondary characteristic of pulmonary stenosis is thickening of the right ventricular anterior wall.

Points of Caution:

1. On the basis of Figure 4-22, it seems probable that a fairly long strip of pulmonary valve needs to be recorded in order to see the abnormally increased presystolic posterior motion of the pulmonary valve. Weyman *et al.*'s criteria apply only to the maximal presystolic posterior motion.

2. The sign is not foolproof, for patients can have significant pulmonary stenosis and not have demonstrated increased posterior presystolic motion.

3. Although it has not been commented on, if infundibular stenosis is also present, the sign probably would not exist.

4. Multiple pulmonary valve diastolic lines may occur in normals. In contrast, multiple diastolic lines occur only occasionally in the normal aortic valves.

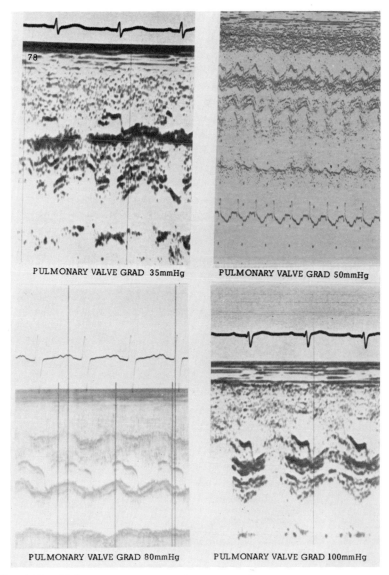

Fig. 4-21.—Pulmonary stenosis. This group of 4 patients was selected for presentation to demonstrate that signs do not always work well. The 4 panels contain echocardiograms of the pulmonary valve in children who have isolated pulmonary valvular stenosis with normal pulmonary artery pressures. None has an impressive A dip. This illustration was shown to Dr. Feigenbaum, who suggested that the presystolic posterior motion was a large percentage of the total posterior excursion in the right upper and lower panels. The lower left panel has been confirmed as a pulmonary valve. Extraneous time lines are present.

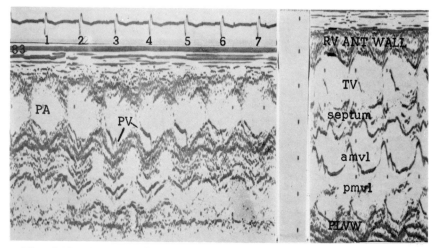

Fig. 4-22.—Severe pulmonary stenosis, gradient 100 mm Hg. This echocardiogram was selected to demonstrate that the posterior presystolic motion can be variable. Note the variability of the presystolic posterior motion, which is maximal just prior to beat 2, less in beat 3 and almost nonexistent in other beats. The right-hand panel demonstrates that the right ventricular wall and septum were both thickened.

5. In the neonate, two leaflets can be seen to open widely in the normal. If the base of a dome were sighted, the same appearance probably would be present in pulmonary stenosis.

6. Increased right ventricular anterior wall thickness accompanies significant pulmonary stenosis. Evaluate the complete echocardiogram.

4.17. Pulmonary Insufficiency
Pertinent literature references: 56, 91.

Isolated pulmonary insufficiency is rare as a congenital anomaly.[163] More often, it is seen in combination with a ventricular septal defect, with or without infundibular or valve ring stenosis. In some cases, pulmonary valve tissue is present but is dysplastic. The pulmonary artery usually is aneurysmally dilated. The right ventricle usually is dilated and may be thickened.

Pulmonary insufficiency acquired secondary to surgery is much more common, especially for tetralogy of Fallot. In these cases, the right ventricle is thickened and may or may not be dilated.

Echocardiographic literature on pulmonary insufficiency is exceedingly sparse. One report states that the tricuspid valve leaflet flutters as does the mitral valve leaflet in aortic insufficiency.[91] This fluttering is alleged to be due to the regurgitant pulmonary insufficiency stream striking the open tricuspid valve leaflet in diastole.

Pulmonary insufficiency can be classified as a cause of right ventricular volume overload.

Our Experience with This Lesion:

Our experience is limited to postoperative tetralogy of Fallot patients in whom we have not seen echocardiographic manifestations of known pulmonary insufficiency. No fluttering of the tricuspid valve leaflet or evidence of right ventricular volume overload have been observed despite efforts to record them. The former may be due to the geographic distance of the tricuspid valve from the pulmonary ring. We believe that the regurgitant stream may strike the right ventricular body first due to the triangular shape of the chamber. This geometry is in contrast to that encountered by the regurgitant aortic insufficiency stream, in which the jet strikes the adjacent anterior mitral valve leaflet in its pathway.

Our inability to demonstrate echographic evidence of right ventricular volume overload may be due to compliance changes brought about by a hypertrophied right ventricular wall in patients with tetralogy of Fallot.

Points of Caution:

1. The absence of tricuspid fluttering and signs of right ventricular volume overload does not mean that the patient does not have pulmonary insufficiency. Much more experience with this lesion is necessary before definitive statements can be made concerning the echocardiographic findings.

2. The echocardiographic findings in primary pulmonary insufficiency with dysplastic or absent pulmonary valve leaflets may be different from the acquired form secondary to operation. Associated cardiac abnormalities and their effects must be taken into account also.

3. Normal tricuspid valves studied with high-resolution equipment seem to flutter a small amount.

4.18-A. Tricuspid Stenosis

Pertinent literature references: 46, 50, 56, 118.

Tricuspid stenosis is a rare congenital entity. Isolated tricuspid stenosis is even less common. The usual differential is between tricuspid stenosis and tricuspid atresia. In the adult, tricuspid stenosis is more common due to longstanding rheumatic disease and nearly always coexists with mitral and/or aortic disease.

The echocardiographic pattern of tricuspid stenosis in adults is similar to the pattern of mitral stenosis. The E – F slope of the stenotic tricuspid valve ranges from 8 to 30 mm/sec.[118]

Our Experience with This Lesion:

We have seen two cases of congenital tricuspid stenosis, one isolated and one in association with pulmonary valvular stenosis. Echoes were performed preoperatively and postoperatively in the patient with a combination tricuspid and pulmonary stenosis and postoperatively in the patient with isolated tricuspid stenosis.

The preoperative echocardiogram in the patient with the combination pulmonary and tricuspid stenosis showed no motion of the tricuspid valve and was not separable from studies of tricuspid atresia, where no valvular motion can be appreciated. Postoperatively, this patient has had echocardiographically demonstrated tricuspid valvular motion, but the amplitude of motion is decreased. The quality of motion was normal.

The postoperative echocardiogram in the patient with isolated tricuspid stenosis shows normal tricuspid valve motion. This patient has had postoperative cardiac catheterization, which showed a decrease in the end diastolic pressure gradient across the tricuspid valve from 19 to 4 mm Hg.

Points of Caution:

1. Absence of the tricuspid valve echo may occur in very severe tricuspid stenosis or in atresia.

2. If the tricuspid valve motion cannot be found, the diagnosis is one of exclusion and therefore has all the problems associated therewith. Multicrystal echo may be of help with this differential.

3. Tricuspid stenosis rarely exists as a single lesion. In the child with congenital tricuspid stenosis, other lesions should be suspected; in the adult with rheumatic tricuspid stenosis, mitral stenosis and aortic stenosis may coexist.

4. Markedly varying E – F slopes can be recorded from the same tricuspid valve.

4.18-B. Tricuspid Atresia

Pertinent literature references: 153, 158.

Tricuspid atresia is a relatively uncommon lesion that is characterized by absence of the tricuspid valve, dilatation of the left ventricle and variable hypoplasia of the right ventricle. An atrial septal defect always is present. A ventricular septal defect occurs in most, but a few patients have the left-to-right shunt at the ductal level. One major paper has been written on this lesion by Meyer and Kaplan.[153]

They indicate that in tricuspid atresia the right ventricle is small, the tricuspid valve echo is absent and the left ventricular cavity is somewhat dilated. These findings are in keeping with the known anatomy. Mitral valve depth is normal in tricuspid atresia. Tricuspid atresia is mentioned elsewhere[158] but not commented on extensively.

Our Experience with This Lesion:

We have had the opportunity to study a few patients with tricuspid atresia. We concur with Meyer and Kaplan's findings. The most difficult problem is proving the absence of the tricuspid valve. The tricuspid valve is relatively easy to find in almost all patients, but in a few it can be quite difficult. We had one patient who had tricuspid stenosis and hypoplasia of the right ventricular cavity. In that patient, we were able to detect no tricuspid valve motion. This was true because the valve was immobilized by the extreme stenosis. The cavity was not detected because it was severely hypoplastic. The patient was operated on and the stenosis relieved. Two years later he still is doing well. Had he been classified as having tricuspid atresia, the wrong surgery would have been performed.

Points of Caution:

1. A considerable effort must be made to find the right ventricular cavity and tricuspid valve before declaring them to be atretic or extremely hypoplastic. This is an instance in which the electrocardiogram is helpful. If left axis deviation and left ventricular hypertrophy are present, a diagnosis of tricuspid atresia is more likely than stenosis.

2. The left atrium and left ventricle may be somewhat larger than normal.

3. The outflow tract of the right ventricle may be visible echocardiographically. This does not rule against the diagnosis of tricuspid atresia.

4.19. Ebstein's Anomaly

Pertinent literature references: 32, 56, 84, 138, 141, 145, 163, 217.

Ebstein's anomaly is characterized by an abnormal origin of one leaflet of the tricuspid valve. Redundant valvular tissue is common. The septal and posterior tricuspid valve leaflets are at varying depths on the right ventricular or septal wall. Leaflet adherence to the right ventricular wall or septum causes the downward displacement of the valve. The farther the adherence the greater the "atrialization" of what should be the right ventricular cavity. Embryologically, an undermining or unpeeling process should take place when the tricuspid valve tissue is liberated from the right ventricular wall. Ebstein's anomaly is thought to result from incomplete undermining of the septal and posterior tricuspid leaflet.[163] Thus, attachments can occur at varying distances from the annulus. In the embryo, the septal and posterior leaflets separate later than the anterior leaflet. This may account for the observation that the anterior leaflet usually is separated in Ebstein's anomaly.[163]

The principal echocardiographic finding in Ebstein's anomaly is delayed tricuspid valve closure with respect to mitral valve closure. Crews et al.[32] used simultaneous phonocardiography and echocardiography to show that delayed tricuspid valve closure coincided with an abnormally wide splitting of S_1. Lundström[141] found delayed tricuspid valve closure and decreased E – F tricuspid valve closure velocity in all 19 of his patients with Ebstein's anomaly. The tricuspid valve echo was also found to have an abnormally anterior position during all of diastole. Examination of septal motion indicated that 1 patient had normal motion, 5 had Type A paradoxical motion and 13 had Type B motion. He also noted that the tricuspid valve echo was displaced more to the left than normal. In a letter to the editor concerning Lundström's article, Kotler[138] agreed that the tricuspid valve amplitude was increased but stated that the tricuspid diastolic closure rate (E – F slope) was normal in 4 of his 6 patients. The terminal closure velocity (B slope) was increased. He and Lundström concluded that some of the differences probably are due to the extreme variability of pathologic expression of the anomaly but that delayed closure and increased closure velocity in patients with great tricuspid amplitude generally were constant findings.

Our Experience with This Lesion:

We have patients with Ebstein's anomaly in whom echocardiography was very helpful. One presented at 1 day of age with cyanosis, a tricuspid insufficiency murmur and a quadruple rhythm. On chest x-ray, cardiomegaly and decreased pulmonary blood flow were noted. An electrocardiogram showed complete right bundle-branch block with right axis deviation. Echocardiography showed delayed tricuspid valve closure, increased tricuspid valve amplitude and a rapid A – C slope (Fig. 4-23). The echocardiogram also showed a normal pulmonary valve, allowing us to at least be sure that the valve was present. Catheterization was avoided. The patient was treated conservatively and improved markedly over 1 week. Her cyanosis decreased and her heart size became smaller as pulmonary vascular resistance dropped.

In older patients, we have noted that echocardiography of the left

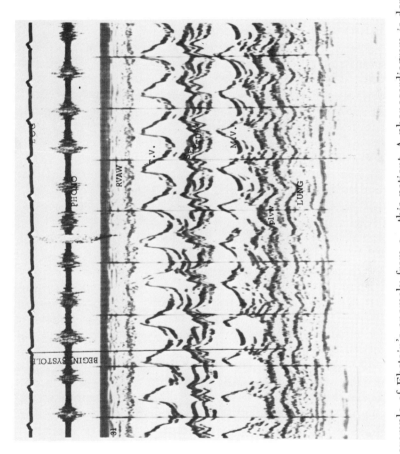

Fig. 4-23.—An example of Ebstein's anomaly from a newborn. Note that the tricuspid leaflet remains open following systole. Direction of septal motion is normal in this patient. A phonocardiogram is demonstrated above the echocardiogram and above that is a somewhat flattened electrocardiogram.

heart can be difficult because of displacement by the huge right atrium.

In general, we agree with the experience of others.

Points of Caution:

1. View the tricuspid valve in the same plane as the mitral valve to establish closure timing.

2. With each echocardiographic examination, seek out the pulmonary valve, as severe pulmonary stenosis or atresia can clinically mimic Ebstein's anomaly in the newborn.

3. In a patient with increased tricuspid valve amplitude, the mitral valve amplitude may seem small. Quantitatively measure each.

4. In Ebstein's anomaly, the tricuspid valve is displaced more to the left than in normals and paradoxical septal motion can be noted. The same findings can occur in any form of right ventricular volume overload.

5. This anomaly has varying degrees of expressivity and so will its echo manifestations.

6. Sometimes the anterior chamber is so large, the left heart may be extremely difficult to find.

4.20. Prosthetic Valves

Pertinent literature references: 12, 56, 75, 76, 111, 112, 114, 146, 147, 168, 172, 175, 181, 200, 206, 207, 231, 240.

Synthetic valve prostheses are of two basic types. First is a caged ball and second is a disk that floats in a cage or is hinged at various positions in the cage. Prosthetic valves have been implanted in children in all ring locations. As some pediatric patients have prosthetic valves, comments about usefulness of echocardiography in following these children are in order.

The major problems with prostheses are thrombus formation, tissue ingrowth, infection,[200] paravalvular leaking, ball variance, improper profile prosthetic valve choice[168] and growth of the heart exceeding the valve's capacity for flow (size limitation).[12]

Echocardiography demonstrates the prosthetic valves especially well in the mitral site and less well in the aortic site.[56] Nanda *et al.*[168] assessed the left ventricular outflow size to assist in mitral selection. They showed that a low-profile prosthesis is desirable when the left ventricular outflow width is less than 20 mm. The outflow was defined as the distance between the left ventricular septal surface and the anterior mitral valve leaflet at the beginning of systole. When a high-profile Starr-Edwards prosthesis was used in patients with left ventricular outflow tracts of less than 20 mm, death occurred in 5 of 7 patients. When a low-profile valve was used in similar patients, 1 of 7 died.

Intraoperatively, Johnson et al.[112] used a gas-sterilized ultrasonic transducer placed on the right ventricular wall and coupled to the right ventricle with saline in order to assess the immediate postoperative prosthetic valve function.

Postoperatively, patients have been serially followed to assess the change in valve function associated with thrombus.[111, 172, 231]

One case report discussed detection of fungal vegetations at the base of the ball valve.[200] The ball moved normally and, at autopsy, the fungal mass was found at the base of the valve but did not involve the struts.

Variance of the ball valve was studied by Johnson et al.[114] by following ball valve size.

Mitral prosthetic valve echoes are markedly visible by echo. The characteristic mitral motion is an anteroposterior movement of the struts and cage coupled with a systolic-diastolic movement of the ball or disk within the first movement (Fig. 4-24). The ball stays open during all of diastole and if it were a mitral valve leaflet it would appear to have a decreased E–F slope. The ball or disk should have a full excursion within its cage. If its movement is incomplete within its chamber, obstruction should be suspected. Normal values for various prosthetic excursions have been generated.[76, 111, 114, 240]

Many prostheses are made of silastic, which has an acoustic velocity of 980 m/sec. Accordingly, the ball will appear very large (Fig. 4-24), since the echographs are set for a velocity of about 1540 m/sec. The ball of the Starr-Edwards prosthesis appears to protrude beyond the sewing ring because of the velocity differential. On the other hand, metal balls will show only the first surface encountered because little sound energy passes through them.

It is important to align the transducer with the ball motion. This can be done by moving the transducer until the opening and closing slopes of the poppet are equal.

Paravalvular leaks will be manifest indirectly by proximal chamber dilatation. Valve obstruction, however, may cause the same indirect sign.

Paravalvular leaks cause two valve motions, one of the ball and the other of the cage. The motions are in different directions, with the ball moving within the cage. The cage, on the other hand, is unhinged and flicks by the transducer quickly. It may be very difficult to track either motion because of the extent of cage swing.

Aortic valve prosthetic motion is much more difficult to assess, as

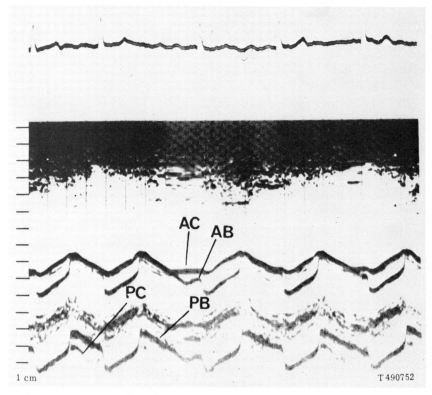

Fig. 4-24. — Starr-Edwards prosthetic valve — echocardiographic representation. *AC* = anterior cage; *PC* = posterior cage; *AB* = anterior ball; *PB* =
posterior ball. The ball appears to move behind its cage, but this is an echocardiographic artifact due to differing velocities of sound in these structures.
This patient had atrial fibrillation, which accounts for differing diastolic
times. (This photograph was modified, with permission, from H. Feigenbaum.[56])

the valve moves in a superior-inferior direction. The best echographic approach is to place the transducer in a supraclavicular space to
the right of the midline and point the beam inferiorly and to the left.
Because of supervening lung tissue, this is not possible in all patients. The suprasternal notch approach has not been discussed for
tracking the aortic valve but may have some merit.

It seems logical that patients with prosthetic valves should be followed serially. Further work is necessary to prove the usefulness of
these echographic techniques but they seem quite promising.

Our Experience with Prosthetic Valves:
Our echocardiographic experience with prosthetic valves in children is limited and no comment is in order.

4.21. Tetralogy of Fallot and Truncus Arteriosus

Pertinent literature references: 26, 56, 103, 220.

These two lesions share some echocardiographic features. The first is discontinuity of the septum and anterior aortic wall. This discontinuity is due to displacement of the aorta with respect to the septum. Common terminology for displacement is "overriding of the aorta." This misalignment and ventricular septal defect are present in both conditions. In truncus arteriosus, the embryologic problem is failure of formation of the spiral septum, and in tetralogy of Fallot the problem is maldivision of the primitive truncus arteriosus, resulting in hypoplasia of the outflow tract of the right ventricle. Patients with tetralogy have a pulmonary artery that is separate from the aorta. A remnant of the pulmonary valve is normally present. Continuity is present between the mitral annulus and the posterior aortic wall.

One type of tetralogy, the "pseudotruncus," lacks a pulmonary valve and frequently the main pulmonary artery is an atretic strand. The difference between a pseudotruncus and a truncus is that in the former group the atretic pulmonary artery arises from the right ventricle whereas in the latter group the pulmonary artery or arteries emerge from the truncus or may be totally absent. Thus, the echocardiographic appearance of pseudotruncus and truncus arteriosus will be similar. On the other hand, the detection of a pulmonary valve in a patient who has discontinuity of the septum and anterior aortic wall indicates that the patient has tetralogy of Fallot.[26]

Second, patients with tetralogy of Fallot demonstrate secondary characteristics, which include an enlarged aorta, a thickened septum, a thickened right ventricular anterior wall and occasionally an enlarged right ventricle. Patients with systemic pulmonary anastomosis or acyanotic tetralogy of Fallot or types of truncus arteriosus with increased pulmonary blood flow may have left ventricular and left atrial enlargement as well. Patients with truncus arteriosus or pseudotruncus have no pulmonary valve and display similar secondary findings. These patients have anatomic mitral aortic continuity.

Our Experience with These Lesions:
Demonstration of septal-aortic discontinuity is relatively easy (Fig. 4-25). One problem that can occur is that the closure line of the aortic or truncal valve can be mistaken for the anterior aortic wall and

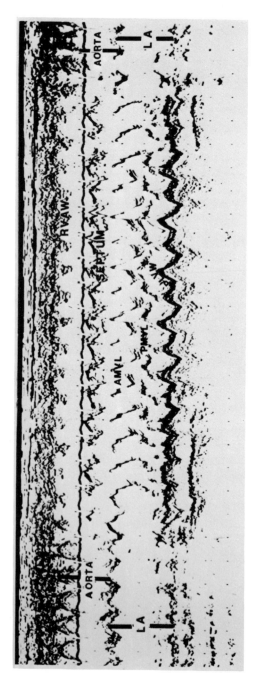

Fig. 4.25.—Tetralogy of Fallot. On the left side of the echocardiogram, the aorta is seen clearly straddling the septum. The posterior wall of the aorta is in clear continuity with the anterior mitral valve leaflet. The right ventricular anterior wall is thickened. The echocardiographer swept back to the aorta on the right side of the panel. This time, the posterior wall of the aorta is not in clear continuity with the anterior mitral leaflet. The systolic levels of the aorta and the leaflet are different. Is the continuity lost? Continuity and lack of continuity are not as clear cut as one might wish.

give the appearance of some degree of continuity. The latter may seem to be easy to rule out, but it can be confusing. To avoid this problem, the full cusp motion of the aortic or truncal valve must be visualized and the anterior vessel wall must be obvious.

Right ventricular anterior wall hypertrophy usually is easy to demonstrate. The body of the right ventricular cavity may be enlarged in the patient with tetralogy, but the cavity of the outflow tract may be quite narrow.

Demonstration of the pulmonary valve in tetralogy clearly is difficult. This is not surprising, since examination of some patients with tetralogy at surgery or autopsy shows that the valve can be miniscule, virtually nonmobile and bicuspid. The valve may be functionally closed in some patients with operatively created aortic-pulmonary shunts. However, if the pulmonary valve is demonstrable and the previously mentioned features are present, the diagnosis of tetralogy is relatively safe. If the pulmonary valve cannot be found, the differentiation of tetralogy of Fallot, truncus and pseudotruncus is not possible by single crystal echocardiography.

The size of the right pulmonary artery can be of considerable importance if a Blalock or Waterston shunt is considered. The size of this vessel can be measured by the suprasternal echocardiographic approach.[81] This measurement has proved helpful in some individuals.

Tetralogy and truncus patients frequently have right aortic arches. In many patients, the presence of a right aortic arch can be determined by suprasternal echocardiography. The details of this approach are covered in Chapter 5.

Patients with tetralogy of Fallot who have operative creation of a left-to-right shunt will have an increase in left atrial size. Details of how the left atrium behaves in the presence of a left-to-right shunt at the ductal level are covered in the section concerned with patent ductus' arteriosus. (See Section 4.2.)

Postoperatively, the patched ventricular septal defect usually aligns the septum with the anterior aortic wall. However, the aorta still will appear large. The patch may be visible on the echocardiogram (Fig. 4-26). The right ventricular hypertrophy frequently remains for years. Although pulmonary insufficiency frequently is present, we have failed to observe the predicted paradoxical septal motion of right ventricular volume overload.

Points of Caution:

1. Be certain that both walls of the aorta are identified and that there is a clear view of the septum. To avoid the possibility that the

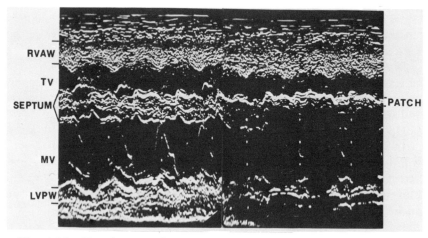

Fig. 4-26. — Tetralogy with patch. Two Polaroid echocardiograms are mounted together. These were taken by stopping the transducer during a sweep for the first and continuing photography with the second. The patch is demonstrated at the right as a relatively thinner area than the septum. Patch motion should not be expected to be normal, and frequently it is paradoxical.

diastolic line of the truncal or aortic valve would be confused with the anterior aortic wall, record the entire valve motion and demonstrate that the diastolic closure line is inside the aorta.

2. Do not assume that failure to record the pulmonary valve means that the patient has a truncus or a pseudotruncus. The valve may not be patent, or may be very small or nonmobile in tetralogy.

3. If right and left arches are to be distinguished by suprasternal echocardiography, the echocardiographer needs considerable experience with known arches before diagnosing an unknown.

4. Do not be satisfied with one demonstration of septal-aortic discontinuity. Apparent discontinuity can be induced by transducer location in normal patients.

5. A truncus arteriosus or tetralogy patient with a normal size aorta is uncommon. Any patient who has this diagnosis and a normal size aorta should be studied carefully.

6. Patients with marked aortic root dilatation secondary to aortic insufficiency or with marked right ventricular enlargement may have apparent but false positive aortic septal discontinuity.

7. Clearly view the right ventricular anterior wall for definition of hypertrophy.

4.22. D-Transposition of the Great Vessels (Situs Solitus)

Pertinent literature references: 24, 42, 87, 103, 106, 128, 197.

The aorta and the pulmonary artery have abnormal positions and ventricular origins in patients with d-transposition of the great vessels and situs solitus. The aorta is anterior, arises from the right ventricular cavity and no longer is in continuity with an atrioventricular valve. The pulmonary artery arises from the left ventricle, is posterior and is in continuity with the anterior mitral valve leaflet. Both semilunar valves are in slightly abnormal locations and usually are aligned in the Z axis. The aortic valve is to the right and the pulmonary valve is to the left and inferior to its usual position. Associated cardiac lesions, such as atrial or ventricular septal defects, are necessary to permit survival.

Gramiak and co-workers[87] described echocardiographic demonstration of d-transposition by transducer location while recording semilunar valves. If the anterior valve was sighted in the usual position of the aortic valve (to the right) and the posterior valve was sighted in the usual position of the pulmonary valve (to the left), the authors stated that d-transposition could be diagnosed.

Dillon et al.[42] demonstrated that if the transducer was pointed directly posteriorly and placed at the fourth left interspace, both semilunar valves could be seen simultaneously in patients with d-transposition. They indicated that this great vessel relationship does not occur in normal children (Fig. 4-27).

Continuity of the posterior semilunar valve and posterior vessel is not helpful in the diagnosis of d-transposition, for it occurs in normals and in patients with d-transposition. Single crystal echocardiography at this time cannot differentiate the fact that the great vessel that is connected to the mitral valve is a pulmonary artery in transposition and an aorta in the normal.

Since the pulmonary semilunar valve opens first, simultaneous timing of the opening of the two semilunar valves may be of importance. Hirschfeld et al.[106] have recorded systolic times (q-semilunar closure interval) in normals and in patients with d-transposition of the great vessels. The pulmonary valve always opened earlier and closed later than the aortic valve. Their results appear to confirm the concept of valve identification by timing when pulmonary resistance is normal.

New techniques for identification of d-transposition[103, 197] have been reported and these are covered in Chapter 7.

Our Experience with This Lesion:

The transducer angulation technique for great vessel orientation is

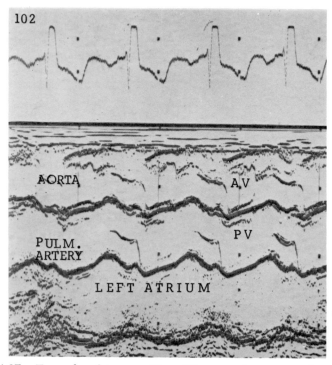

Fig. 4-27.—Example of transposition. The transducer was placed at the fourth left interspace and aimed directly posteriorly. Both the anterior aortic valve and the posterior pulmonary valve could be visualized simultaneously. A similar picture can be obtained in children with dilated pulmonary arteries without transposition and in normal children when the transducer is higher on the chest and aimed inferiorly. The pulmonary valve opens earlier and closes about the same time in the illustration.

very difficult to perform reliably. It often is easier to document normal great vessel orientation by this technique than to make the diagnosis of d-transposition. Additionally, differences in angulation between the two vessels may be too subtle for easy detection. Perhaps we have not mastered this technique, but clearly it is difficult to apply with the single beam echocardiogram. On the other hand, we have been able to sight both semilunar valves simultaneously from the fourth left interspace in most, but not all, of our patients with d-transposition. In most instances, the latter technique was diagnostic. However, we have had false positives in normal infants in some instances when semilunar valves were simultaneously sighted from the fourth left interspace with the transducer held precisely as Dillon indicated. This was particularly true if the patient had dilatation of the pulmonary artery. Simultaneous sighting of both semilunar valves in the normal is also enhanced when a large-diameter transducer is used. This produces a wider beam than the 6-mm probes. Simultaneous recording of the valves should be accepted only when the narrow beam is used.

The relative time of opening of the two semilunar valves needs more evaluation. It may be useful, but the effect of other lesions on valve dynamics must be worked out.

Secondary features of d-transposition include thickened right ventricular anterior wall and frequently a dilated left atrium and ventricle if the left-to-right shunt is large.

Points of Caution:

1. The most important point regarding simultaneous sighting of the semilunar valves is the precision with which the transducer must be located at the fourth left interspace and directed posteriorly. A slight shift of the transducer superiorly with a slight inferior rightward aim will demonstrate simultaneous semilunar valves in most normal infants.

2. Localization of semilunar valves by direction of the transducer and depth of the valve is treacherous. We have tried this numerous times and have been frustrated by usually finding that the valves are sighted simultaneously.

3. Not all children with d-transposition have semilunar valves that can be recorded simultaneously after the method of Dillon. One child with d-transposition who was studied repeatedly had the pulmonary valve slightly to the left but elevated enough to prevent simultaneous sighting. Moreover, the valve was so little leftward that the transducer angulation technique also was not helpful.

4. Occasionally, normal children can have simultaneous semilunar valves recorded from the fourth left interspace.

5. Simultaneous semilunar valve technique is not particularly easy. It may require considerable time and effort. The reason that this is true is that the valves and vessels are not precisely aligned in the Z axis. We have found that most of the time that we have spent examining babies for this criterion has been used to be absolutely certain that the simultaneous structures that we saw were truly semilunar valves. If they were perfectly aligned, simultaneous sighting would be easier. Usually, however, one can record only one cusp of each valve at a time.

6. It may be possible to locate the positions of the atrioventricular and aortic and pulmonary valves in order to map out complex cardiac

abnormalities even in malpositions. In our experience, this is most difficult to do reliably and is more amenable to cross-sectional echo techniques (see Chapter 7).

4.23. Double Outlet Right Ventricle

Pertinent literature references: 24, 25, 170, 171.

The double outlet right ventricle is an infrequent congenital cardiac abnormality that, in part, is characterized by displacement of the aorta and presence of a ventricular septal defect. Two major types are recognized. In one, the ventricular septal defect is related to the aorta and in the other the ventricular septal defect is related to the pulmonary artery. An anatomic spectrum of great vessel relationships exists between the two forms. The precise alignment of the great vessels varies from patient to patient, but usually the semilunar valves are aligned in the Y and Z coordinates. Since both vessels originate from the right ventricle, mitral-semilunar (aortic or pulmonic) continuity should be broken as the ventricular septal defect is interposed between the valves. Although this usually is true, in some patients a rather long anterior mitral valve leaflet reaches to or almost through the ventricular septal defect and appears to be, or actually is, in continuity with a semilunar valve.[170]

Chesler et al.[24, 25] reported discontinuity of the mitral valve and aortic annulus that was distinguishable by echocardiography in patients with double outlet right ventricle. They related the depth of the anterior mitral valve leaflet in systole to the depth of the aortic posterior wall. A double outlet right ventricle was said to be present if the depth of these two structures were different. Moreover, they reported that actual echocardiographic discontinuity of the structures was recognizable. This discontinuity usually appeared as a break during the sweep from the mitral to the aortic valve. To date, the publication by Chesler et al.[25] is the only major echocardiographic investigation of this lesion.

Our Experience with This Lesion:

The systolic depth of the anterior mitral valve leaflet is not directly related to the posterior aortic wall depth in some normal children and in some with heart disease. Thus, this criterion lacks differentiation capability.

Mitral-aortic continuity has seemed to be present in some of our patients with catheterization and operatively proved double outlet right ventricle (Fig. 4-28). The apparent continuity occurs echocardiographically because of the arrangement of the aorta, the ventricular septal defect and the mitral valve. The mitral attachment is very close

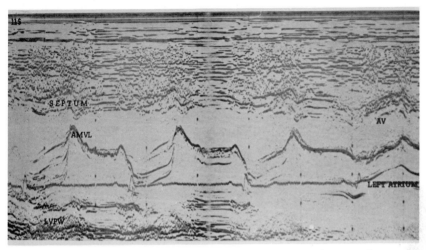

Fig. 4-28.—Example of a double outlet right ventricle in a 2-year-old child. Diagnosing a double outlet right ventricle can be very treacherous by single crystal echocardiography. This echocardiogram demonstrates continuity of the septum with the anterior wall of a great vessel that was presumed to be the aorta, and the mitral valve appears to be continuous with the posterior wall. Some echoes are seen below the aorta, the origin of which is not known. A semilunar valve appears inside the great vessel. At operation, this child had double outlet right ventricle. The mitral valve was excessively long and protruded through the ventricular septal defect.

to the aortic root in some patients with double outlet right ventricle. In that group, it might not be possible to detect discontinuity by single crystal echocardiography. However, in some patients with double outlet right ventricle, the alignment clearly produces discontinuity. Thus, all patients with double outlet right ventricles do not have the echocardiographic disruption of mitral-aortic continuity. Further, all patients who seem to have discontinuity do not have double outlet right ventricle. One group of patients who have apparent lack of mitral-aortic continuity are those with very dilated left ventricles as the result of a myopathic process. These patients may have a marked depth differential between the mitral valve anterior leaflet in systole and the posterior aortic wall. A carefully performed sweep reveals anatomic continuity. This entity represents one of the important echocardiographic differentials for double outlet right ventricle.

Secondary characteristics of double outlet right ventricle should be sought echocardiographically. If the left-to-right shunt is large, the patient would be expected to have a large left atrium and ventricle.

The pulmonary and aortic valve may appear slightly displaced; however, the displacement is not diagnostic. Right ventricular hypertrophy is uniform. If the ventricular septal defect is small, ventricular obstruction may be present, which will produce left ventricular hypertrophy. The aorta lacks its normal posterior sweep, and simultaneous visualization of the anterior and posterior aortic wall at the aortic root often is impossible because the walls begin at different levels in the Y coordinate. The transducer must be directed more cephalad to see the anterior aortic wall. The posterior aortic wall is relatively easy to find in this lesion.

Points of Caution:

1. The systolic depth of the mitral valve may not align with the systolic depth of the posterior aorta in normals or in patients with other cardiac lesions.

2. A few patients with double outlet right ventricles have unquestionable mitral-aortic continuity by echocardiography; others have neither mitral-aortic nor mitral-pulmonic continuity.

3. Patients with dilated left ventricles and no double outlet right ventricle may have apparent mitral aortic discontinuity, but a very carefully performed slow sweep from the mitral valve to the aortic ring usually will reveal continuity.

4. Single crystal, single dimension echocardiography probably is not the best answer to echocardiographic diagnosis of the double outlet right ventricle. This lesion is covered in more detail in Chapter 7, which deals with newer echocardiographic techniques.

4.24. Hypoplastic Left Heart

Pertinent literature references: 6, 24, 145, 153, 213.

Diagnosis of patients with hypoplastic left heart syndrome is an important use of echocardiography. The anatomy of this syndrome is quite variable. Most commonly, one of the two left-sided valves is atretic and the left ventricle is hypoplastic. The aorta and its valve may be atretic, small or normal in size. A number of publications have appeared in which 1 to 6 patients with hypoplastic left heart syndrome have been studied. Meyer and Kaplan[153] reviewed echocardiograms of 6 children with hypoplastic left hearts. Diagnostic features included an enlarged right ventricular cavity with a dimension of 2.38–3.2 cm. The left ventricular cavity was small, with a dimension of 0.4–0.9 cm. The mitral valve echo was absent or poorly visualized. Mitral valve depth appeared to be normal. Lundström and Edler[145] corroborated the finding of absent or decreased mitral valve amplitude. Solinger *et al.*[213] indicated that the mobility of the ante-

rior leaflet of the mitral valve and ring was less than 50% of normal
in their 2 patients with hypoplastic mitral valves. Chesler and co-
workers[24] reported 1 patient with gross hypoplasia of the left heart,
but this patient also had other findings that are atypical of hypoplastic
left hearts, such as polysplenia.

Our Experience with This Lesion:

For unexplained reasons, hypoplastic left heart syndrome is relatively uncommon in Arizona. We have had the opportunity to study
only 4 patients with this condition. We had little difficulty in recognizing hypoplastic left heart by using the criteria of Meyer (Fig. 4-29).
In all instances, the left ventricle was so small and the valves so
hypoplastic that we had no differential problem. If the cavity or valve
opening is relatively small, normal data could be used in a statistical
fashion to determine the possibility of hypoplastic left heart syn-

Fig. 4-29.—Example of hypoplastic left heart. Note the small annular
motion of the hypoplastic mitral valve. The left ventricle and septum could
not be echocardiographically demonstrated in this patient. At autopsy, mitral
atresia and a slit left ventricular cavity were present.

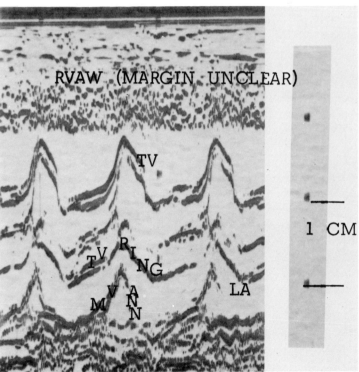

drome. In that instance, mitral amplitude, left ventricular cavity size, aortic valve opening and the size of the aortic root could be compared to the normal fifth percentile data. It is apparent that 4% of normal children have values less than the fifth percentile and therefore a degree of judgment will have to be utilized.

Points of Caution:

1. Mitral valve motion may be decreased in patients with myocarditis, but in that lesion the left ventricle is dilated. This should not offer a considerable differential problem.

2. Right ventricular volume overload can increase the size of the right ventricle and make the left ventricle appear small by comparison.

3. Rarely, a tumor can fill the left ventricular cavity and give an illusion of a hypoplastic left ventricle. A right ventricular tumor has been reported that displaced the septum posteriorly, compressing the left ventricle to half normal size.[6]

4. Single ventricle can be confused with a hypoplastic left or hypoplastic right ventricle; however, the mitral valve and the aortic valve usually have normal amplitude in this condition.

5. Patients with severe aortic stenosis or coarctation of the aorta may have markedly thickened left ventricular and septal walls and the cavity may appear small (Fig. 4-7). These children are salvageable and the echocardiogram should not be confused with that of a true hypoplastic left heart.

6. Occasionally, when only a slitlike left ventricular cavity is present, it may not be identified echocardiographically. In such patients, the differentiation of hypoplastic left heart from single ventricle may be difficult, especially when the origin of the diminutive aorta is not clear. This may also occur if the septum is rotated into a plane parallel to the incident sound energy and is not imaged adequately (Fig. 4-29).

4.25. Right Ventricular Hypertrophy

Pertinent literature reference: 230.

Right ventricular hypertrophy is defined as excessive thickness of the right ventricle by comparison with normal standards. The echocardiographic literature is virtually void of information concerning the right ventricular anterior wall and right ventricular hypertrophy. This probably is due to the fact that clear visualization of the right ventricle is difficult with standard techniques and transducers, but it can be evaluated relatively easily with high-frequency transducers and the techniques detailed in Chapter 5. Right ventricular anterior wall thickness is measured at the beginning of the QRS in the plane that simultaneously demonstrates the posterior leaflet of the mitral valve. Little normal information is available in the literature regarding this structure. Our normal data are in Chapter 3.

Our Experience with This Lesion:

Our normal data for the right ventricular wall thickness show that only trivial growth occurs with age. The right ventricular wall was measured to the nearest half millimeter to determine normal standards. After the first 2 months of life, right ventricular wall thickness did not exceed 3.5 mm in any normal patients living at an altitude of 2500 feet above sea level.

In our experience, hypertrophy occurs most commonly when the right ventricle must generate excessive pressure in order to overcome right ventricular infundibular or pulmonary valvular stenosis or pulmonary vascular or parenchymal disease. We would anticipate that prevalence data for individuals living at higher altitudes might show greater right ventricular anterior wall thickness because some will have increased pulmonary artery pressures. We have also occasionally observed right ventricular hypertrophy in patients with lesions that cause sustained high left atrial pressure. On the other hand, it is uncommon to find right ventricular hypertrophy in patients with isolated left-to-right shunts.

Electrocardiographic and echocardiographic correlation is somewhat better for the right ventricular wall than the left. However, this is not true in patients with lung disease or in the newborn. A study of right ventricular anterior wall thickness and clinical severity of cystic fibrosis has yielded a good correlation.[230] The electrocardiogram and vectorcardiogram did not correlate well in this condition. We have consistently observed neonates with anterior or rightward voltage criteria beyond the ninety-fifth percentile who do not show echocardiographic evidence of right ventricular hypertrophy.

It is important to recognize that echocardiography does not measure all portions of the right ventricular wall. The outflow tract in the plane above the aortic valve and the anterior wall at the level of the posterior mitral leaflet can be measured. It is conceivable that a hypertrophied portion of the right ventricular wall might not be measured.

The most severe forms of right ventricular hypertrophy occur in patients with severe pulmonary stenosis, tetralogy of Fallot, transposition and other lesions that require considerable pressure work of the right ventricle. Changes in right ventricular wall thickness probably occur very slowly. Any sudden change must be questioned.

Points of Caution:

1. Do not try to measure right ventricular wall thickness if the wall is not seen clearly.

2. During systole, the right ventricular anterior wall frequently pulls away from the chest wall and creates the illusion of excessive contraction. Measure only at end diastole.

3. If successive measurements of right ventricular wall thickness change by more than a millimeter, consider the possibility that a measurement error has occurred.

4.26. Left Ventricular Hypertrophy

Pertinent literature references: 3, 7, 58, 59, 60, 94, 95, 122, 209, 226.

Left ventricular hypertrophy is defined as an abnormal thickening of the left ventricle wall. It usually is associated with conditions that cause the left ventricle to produce excessive pressure work.

Prior to echocardiography, left ventricular hypertrophy usually was diagnosed or measured in four ways:

1. Angiographically.
2. At autopsy.
3. At the time of surgery.
4. By electrocardiography.

Angiography provided the only actual in-vivo dynamic measurement, but it produced potentially erroneous information because of poor resolution of both surfaces of the ventricle, particularly the epicardium. Autopsy provided a single nondynamic measurement. Dynamic measurement could be performed at operation, but such measurements are difficult because of limited exposure and cardiac irritability. Nondynamic measurements during cardioplegia are simple to obtain but do not truly represent usual end diastolic ventricular wall thickness.

Assessments concerning the presence and severity of hypertrophy most commonly are made by electrocardiography. These criteria include voltage measurements and alterations in the amplitude and direction of the S–T segment and T wave.[95, 122]

Feigenbaum and others have demonstrated that the posterior left ventricular wall and septum can be dynamically measured by echocardiography.[7, 58-60, 209, 226] Feigenbaum found a high correlation between echocardiographic left ventricular posterior wall measurements and measurements made at surgery.[58] Surprisingly, we have found no pediatric studies that correlate electrocardiographic interpretation of hypertrophy and echocardiographic measurements of wall thickness. However, echocardiography has been used to study the left ventricle in disease. Echocardiographic left ventricular wall measurements have been demonstrated to be increased in patients with systemic hypertension.[3]

Our Results with Measurement of Left Ventricular Wall Thickness:

We routinely measure end diastolic ventricular wall thickness and compare the value to normal standards on every child who has an echocardiogram. We have observed only a weak correlation of wall thickness and pediatric electrocardiographic criteria for left ventricular hypertrophy.

1. Wall thickness increases slightly with age and is a highly repeatable measurement (see Chapter 3). Excessive left ventricular wall thickness is common in children with systemic hypertension and aortic valvular stenosis but is distinctly uncommon in patients with left-to-right shunts. If patients with systemic hypertension are treated successfully for their disease or if patients with aortic stenosis are operated on, left ventricular wall thickness usually decreases over a period of months.

Points of Caution in Measuring Left Ventricular Wall Thickness:

1. Wall thickness should be measured from the endocardium to the pericardium, but the thickness of the pericardium should not be included in the measurement. Actually, the pericardium is quite thin, but its echo is relatively bright and can appear to be wide, particularly by the Polaroid technique. Decreasing instrument gain usually will decrease the width of the pericardial echo.

2. Chordae echoes parallel, and may be confused with, the endocardial surface. Such an error would make the left ventricular wall appear too thick.

3. Left ventricular wall thickness always should be measured at the end of diastole in the plane that simultaneously shows the posterior mitral valve leaflet. The transducer should be as perpendicular to the chest wall as possible.

4. Occasionally an error is made by measuring the apical portion of the left ventricle in the area of the papillary muscles. This inclusion of papillary muscle causes the left ventricular posterior wall to appear thicker than if examined in the proper plane.

5. If the left ventricular wall measurement varies more than a millimeter on a day-to-day basis, some measurement error probably is present.

4.27. Increased Left Ventricular End Diastolic Pressure

Pertinent literature reference: 56.

In the normal heart, the D – E slope is rapid and is followed by a smooth, rapid A – C slope. Mitral valve closure begins sooner in patients with decreased left ventricular compliance, causing the A point to occur earlier than normal. Prior to ventricular systole, the left ventricular and left atrial pressures are nearly equal and mitral valve closure is somewhat interrupted, as demonstrated by a plateau between A and C. Mitral valve closure is delayed because it occurs at a higher left ventricular pressure. Thus, the A–C interval is increased. Feigenbaum indicates that the adult normal P–R interval is 0.06 second greater than the A–C interval. In the adult, a (P–R)–(A–C) interval of 0.06 second or less indicates a left ventricular end diastolic pressure of at least 20 mm.

In patients who have a very high initial left ventricular pressure, the mitral valve opens against a high left ventricular end systolic pressure. Thus, the mitral valve D–E slope is diminished. The left ventricle does not fill well because of decreased compliance and therefore a large volume of ventricular filling occurs with atrial contraction. Thus, the amplitude of the A point generally is increased.

Our Experience with This Lesion:
We concur with Feigenbaum's remarks.

4.28. Cardiomyopathy

Pertinent literature references: 56, 77, 157, 195.

Cardiomyopathy signifies intrinsic disease of the cardiac muscle. Coronary artery disease usually is excluded in pediatric cardiology. Cardiomyopathy in pediatric patients includes mainly such conditions as myocarditis, familial abnormalities of the myocardium, storage diseases and fibroelastosis. Very little information has appeared in the echocardiographic literature regarding cardiomyopathy. Feigenbaum[56] stated that it may be difficult to separate patients with cardiomyopathy and ischemic myocardial disease. He showed that cardiac motion in myopathy is reduced and that paradoxical or totally akinetic segments are not present.

Cardiomyopathy may cause secondary mitral regurgitation because of distortion of the mitral valve apparatus by the dilated ventricles. Millward and co-workers[157] indicated that the two mitral valve leaflets never completely approximate each other during ventricular systole, as evidenced by multiple systolic echoes. However, multiple systolic echoes can occur for many reasons and are not diagnostic of mitral insufficiency. Also, they pointed out that the average mitral excursion was decreased in cardiomyopathy (Fig. 4-30). Glaser[77] replied to their publication and indicated that the mitral valve was posteriorly displaced in cardiomyopathy associated with some mitral insufficiency. He demonstrated an echocardiogram showing a

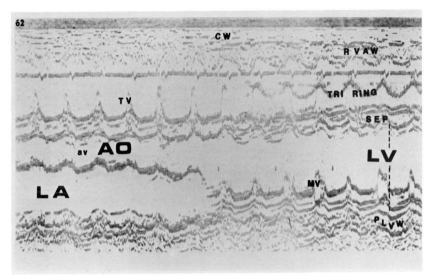

Fig. 4-30. — Myocardiopathy in a 6-month-old child. This photograph shows an impressively large left ventricular cavity with extremely small posteriorly displaced mitral motion. The tricuspid valve and ring are visualized also. Note the sweep from the mitral valve to the aorta. A continuity is demonstrated, but had the sweep been done more quickly, the continuity surely would have been lost.

marked disparity between the level of the posterior aortic root and the systolic portion of the mitral valve. His echocardiogram also displayed decreased mitral valve motion.

Although it might be anticipated that fibroelastosis would be easily sighted by echocardiography, we are not aware of echocardiographic reports in this condition. Similarly, we are not aware of reports of the echocardiographic findings in myocarditis, glycogen storage disease or other myopathies of childhood.

Our Experience with These Lesions:

We agree with Glaser[77] that the mitral valve appears to be posteriorly displaced in cardiomyopathies associated with marked dilatation of the left ventricle. Mitral-aortic continuity is preserved but may be very treacherous to demonstrate. Mitral valve amplitude may be markedly decreased. When the beam is swept from the aorta to the left ventricle, the posterior mitral valve leaflet usually is sighted at the same time as the anterior leaflet. The posterior mitral leaflet may appear to move in a manner almost parallel to the anterior leaflet. This probably is not evidence of mitral stenosis but merely reflects spatial derangement of the papillary muscles during ventricular dilatation. In fact, the same problem may produce the mitral insufficiency in this condition. Posterior left ventricular wall motion in cardiomyopathy may be decreased if mitral insufficiency is minimal or increased if mitral insufficiency is greater. By far the most impressive feature of the cardiomyopathy is the marked ventricular dilatation. The echographic determination of mean Vcf detects decreased myocardial contractility in these patients.

Points of Caution:

1. It seems clear that not enough echocardiographic information is yet available to make conclusions concerning cardiomyopathy.

2. Do not be misled by the difference in depth between the posterior aortic wall and the systolic portion of the mitral motion in cardiomyopathy. There is no double outlet right ventricle in this condition, for continuity is present.

3. Multiple mitral systolic or diastolic lines occur in normals and abnormals.

4. A very complete examination is required, for the patient may have a myocardial infarction as the primary disease. This would be diagnosed by abnormal motion or akinetic segments of the left ventricle.

4.29. Coronary Artery Disease

Pertinent literature references: 18, 21, 31, 67, 68, 78, 108–110, 124, 133, 150, 178, 216.

Coronary artery disease is a very rare problem in children even though coronary artery occlusion, as a result of atherosclerosis, may begin during the childhood years.[53] The most common congenital coronary artery problem in children is anomalous origin of the left coronary artery from the pulmonary artery. A single abstract has been written about this condition and indicates posterior displacement of of the aortic valve and dominance of the anterior cusp.[78] We cannot confirm or deny the conclusions of this abstract.

Since coronary artery disease and its complications are, for all practical purposes, out of the realm of pediatrics and since we have had almost no experience with this condition, we refer the reader to the various publications that deal with this subject in the adult.[18, 21, 31, 67, 68, 108-110, 124, 133, 150, 178, 216]

4.30. Intracardiac Tumors

Pertinent literature references: 6, 49, 51, 56, 66, 73, 80, 84, 122, 136, 148, 184, 188, 189, 199, 208, 242.

Cardiac tumors can be malignant by location; i.e., they can cause fatal rhythm disturbances or can be hemodynamically obstructive. Further, some, especially myxoma, may be embolic or can be a nidus for clot formation. Angiographic procedures and catheter manipulation procedures can dislodge these masses. Thus, a noninvasive detection technique such as echocardiography is especially desirable for these lesions.

The most common intracardiac tumor demonstrated by echocardiography in the adult has been the left atrial myxoma. This is reasonable, since myxoma accounts for 50% of all primary intracardiac tumors. Some right atrial myxomas have also been reported.[56, 84] Myxoma is a less common tumor in the pediatric age group but has been reported in patients as young as 3 years. Gasul et al.[73] found that 5% of the reported 250 cases of myxoma occurred in children.

Tumors found in the neonate include rhabdomyoma, lipoma, hemangioma and malignant sarcoma.[73, 122] These are primarily intraventricular but can be found in the walls, septum or atrial chambers. One intraventricular tumor has been demonstrated by echocardiography in the right ventricle of a neonate[6] that displaced the intraventricular septum posteriorly. The pathologic diagnosis was rhabdomyoma.

Myxomas usually are pedunculated. Their movement is in the direction of blood flow in their respective chambers. The left atrial myxoma is seen as a mass of echoes behind the mitral valve. In diastole, it may pass through the open mitral valve leaflets. Martinez et al.[148] and Feigenbaum[56] stress that a complete echocardiographic evaluation demands three views:

1. The left atrium in the plane of the aortic leaflets.

2. A view of the anterior mitral valve leaflet plane with the left atrium posterior (Fig. 4-31).

3. The plane that subtends both mitral leaflets with the left ventricle posterior.

The posterior mitral valve leaflet echoes in some patients with mitral stenosis occasionally can be confused with tumor. However, in mitral stenosis, these echoes are lost when the echo beam is swept from the left ventricle to the left atrium. Such a sweep would make a tumor more prominent.

The same dynamics exist for right atrial myxomas. In this case, the tumor passes into the right ventricular cavity through the tricuspid valve during diastole. In one case,[84] pronounced paradoxical septal motion was present.

Our Experience with This Lesion:

We have seen no atrial myxomas. The only opportunity we have had to evaluate a tumor is in the infant described previously.[6] Initial-

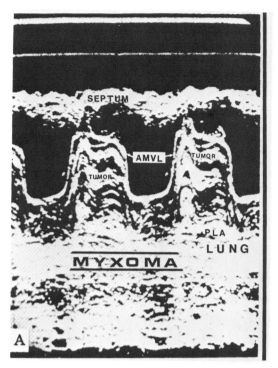

Fig. 4-31.—Left atrial myxoma. The heavy echoes in the position of the mitral valve represent the myxoma. Note that they move anteriorly in diastole. The valve tissue itself is poorly seen anterior to this heavy band of echoes. The posterior left atrial wall is indicated. (Modified, with permission, from H. Feigenbaum.[56])

ly, we believed that he had a hypoplastic left heart, but closer evaluation showed that a mass of echoes persisted from the right ventricular outflow area to the tricuspid area, irrespective of the gain setting. Further, the right ventricular anterior wall moved separately from the mass and a slitlike cavity was present between it and the tumor. The mass appeared to be attached to the septum. When the left ventricular cavity was measured, it was not hypoplastic. The mitral valve had decreased D–E and E–F slopes but otherwise was normal. The aortic valve and aorta were normal.

In centers in which there is a vast echocardiographic experience with tumors, the diagnosis probably can be made safely without catheterization. However, more experience probably will be necessary before the pediatric cardiologist can rely solely on echocardiography for complete diagnosis of cardiac tumors. Multicrystal echocardiography may improve the situation, since more events and areas can be viewed simultaneously.

Points of Caution:

1. When evaluating the infant with a suspected intraventricular tumor, care must be taken to investigate the right ventricular cavity as well as the left, since the tumor may be in either ventricle or on the septum.

2. Echocardiographic technique must be meticulous when evaluating tumors. Insufficient damping or rejection can create a shower of echoes that can be confused with tumor. Too little gain can lead to a false negative.

3. It is difficult to be certain that one is not dealing with a clot, especially in the older patient who may have atrial fibrillation.

4. There is a possibility that right ventricular muscle bundles might be confused with intraventricular tumors.

5. It seems important to follow patients by echo after tumor removal, since some have recurred.

6. Feigenbaum has pointed out that the stenotic posterior mitral valve leaflet with mitral stenosis can be confused with a myxoma. The stenotic posterior leaflet disappears as the beam is directed from the left ventricular cavity into the left atrial cavity. In contrast, myxomas would be more apparent as the beam was directed toward the left atrial cavity. A sweep is necessary during the echocardiographic evaluation.

7. Myxoma can occur in the right atrium and may be small enough to be within the cavity of the right atrium and not pedunculated. These will be missed by echocardiography during routine evaluation. The right atrium receives little echocardiographic attention.

4.31. Disorders of Conduction

Pertinent literature references: 1, 5, 35, 37 – 39, 131, 150.

Disorders of conduction is a topic that could occupy an entire text and exceeds the scope of this one. To date, conduction has received little echocardiographic attention.

Normal cardiac conduction originates in the sino-atrial node, passes through the atria, the atrioventricular node, the bundle of His and thence through three fascicles into the ventricles. Stimulation brings about septal, right ventricular and left ventricular muscle contraction, in that order.

The effects of cardioversion of atrial fibrillation on cardiac function were studied.[35] Left atrial dimension, left ventricular end diastolic dimension and mitral valve motion were evaluated before and 1 hour after the conversion of atrial fibrillation in 21 patients. Mitral A waves appeared after cardioversion, corroborating that they are resultant from atrial contraction. Left atrial dimension decreased and left ventricular end diastolic dimension increased, suggesting increased ejection fraction, stroke volume and cardiac output.

Alderman et al.[5] evaluated 3 patients with atrial flutter. They found an anterior peaking motion of the open mitral valve leaflet or poppet in 1 patient with a prosthetic valve in the region of the nadir of the electrocardiographic atrial flutter wave. The extent of anterior mitral valve peaking was influenced by the volume of left ventricular filling. The left ventricular filling influenced the intensity of atrial flutter sounds, especially the clicking of the prosthetic poppet.

Intraventricular conduction has also gained echocardiographic attention. The echocardiogram in complete right bundle-branch block

Fig. 4-32.—Example of left bundle-branch block. Carotid tracing, phonocardiogram and electrocardiogram are above the echocardiogram. T = transducer interface; S = interventricular septum; PLV = posterior left ventricular wall; M = abnormal onset of motion; P = abnormal peak of motion; N = septal notch; C = abnormal systolic contraction. This figure demonstrates abnormal septal motion in complete left bundle-branch block. This is compared with a normal echocardiogram at the right. (Modified, with permission, from I. G. McDonald and Circulation.[150])

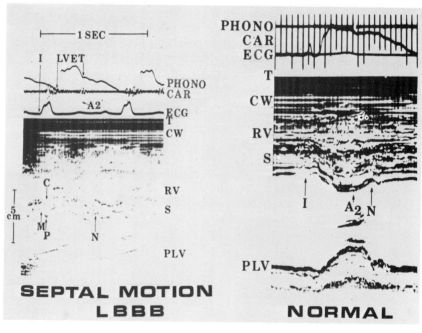

does not differ from normal.[37] Complete left bundle-branch block, on
the other hand, is characterized by a sharp early posterior motion of
the septum, followed by paradoxical septal motion (Fig. 4-32). Right
and left ventricular posterior walls move normally. The initial systolic posterior septal motion is not found in right ventricular volume
overload.[1, 38, 39, 131, 150]

Our Experience with This Lesion:
We agree that the echocardiographic pattern in complete right
bundle-branch block does not differ from normal. Atrial fibrillation or
left bundle-branch block are rare in children, and we have little echocardiographic experience with these problems. Patients with com-

Fig. 4-33. – Effect of a premature ventricular contraction on aortic systolic
duration. This photograph was selected because it demonstrates the need to
quantitate. At first glance, the premature contraction might seem to demonstrate less opening of the aortic valve. In fact, if measured, it can be determined that its opening is the same as the two previous beats. The difference is
one of duration. This has been the usual finding that we have seen with
premature ventricular contractions. Occasionally, the opening may be slightly
less. (The photograph was provided by Dr. Gordon Ewy.)

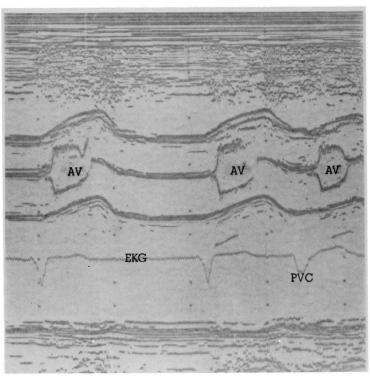

plete heart block demonstrate varying amplitudes of the mitral valve A waves, depending on the relationship of the electrocardiographic P wave to the QRS complex.

Premature ventricular contractions cause variable duration of aortic valve opening, but the intercusp distance usually is unaffected (Fig. 4-33).

Points of Caution:

1. Include high-quality electrocardiogram and time indicators with every echocardiogram to improve correlation of arrhythmias and echo.

2. A clear echo of the septum is necessary for differentiating right ventricular volume overload and complete left bundle-branch block. Observe carefully for the initial septal downstroke.

3. Evaluate not only qualitative measurements but also chamber dimensions and quantitative timing in patients who may have decreased cardiac function as a result of arrhythmia.

4.32. Bacterial Endocarditis

Pertinent literature references: 41, 241.

Bacterial endocarditis is a result of the invasion of cardiac tissue by organisms. Infection usually begins in the low-pressure area of a jet lesion. In the adult, the lesions most commonly are left-sided but in the child many sites are possible. In both groups, nonendothelialized portions of prostheses are common sites.

The most comprehensive echocardiographic review of endocarditis was published by Dillon and co-workers.[41] They demonstrated aortic and mitral valvular vegetations in patients with known endocarditis. In one instance, the echocardiogram instigated the search for the disease. In each instance, autopsy or surgical confirmation was available. They found that the valve leaflets were nonuniformly thickened, and dense shaggy echoes were attached to the leaflets (Fig. 4-34). Vegetations as small as 2 mm were recorded. However, they were unable to find vegetations in all patients with the disease. All valves moved normally despite apparent thickening, and this fact separates the valve afflicted with endocarditis from one that is calcified. In 3 patients with presumed cures, the size and intensity of the echoes increased with time.

Myxomas could be confused with endocarditic lesions, but the former usually is not attached to a valve and is visible within the chamber beyond the area of the valve.

Wise *et al.*[241] published an echocardiogram of a patient with aortic valve endocarditis who showed early closure of the mitral valve.

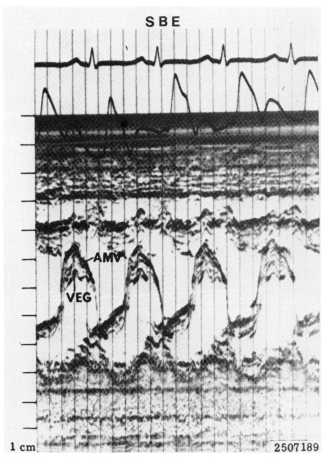

Fig. 4-34.—Example of vegetations. This echogram is from a patient with bacterial endocarditis involving the anterior mitral valve leaflet. There is a heavy band of echoes under the anterior mitral leaflet in diastole. These are originating from the vegetations (*VEG*). (Modified, with permission, from J. C. Dillon *et al.*[41])

They suggested that early closure was due to acutely increased left ventricular end diastolic pressure.

Our Experience with This Lesion:

Our experience is limited to one 6-year-old girl with a small ventricular septal defect. With no antecedent event, she developed clinical findings and culture evidence of bacterial endocarditis. Echocardiography had been performed 6 months prior to admission and was normal. With endocarditis, she had a mass under the septal leaflet of the tricuspid valve on the right septal surface that jutted into the right ventricular cavity during systole. At the end of her hospitalization, the mass no longer was observable. We suspect that this was a vegetation on the right septal surface of a membranous ventricular septal defect. Six months later, the echocardiogram remained normal.

Dillon indicated that vegetations increase in size even after apparent cure. We cannot explain the disappearance of the presumed echo vegetation representation in our patient. Possibly it silently embolized or completely healed.

Points of Caution:

1. Some echographs make normal valves appear shaggy, smeary and thick.

2. Serial follow-up seems necessary.

3. Absence of a characteristic echocardiogram does not mean absence of the disease.

4.33. Pericardial Effusion

Pertinent literature references: 47, 52, 55, 61–64, 72, 82, 107, 112, 134, 154, 164, 174, 187, 188, 189, 194, 214.

Echocardiography probably is the most sensitive technique for detecting pericardial effusion.[154] Radioactive and contrast techniques are less likely to detect small effusions. The safety and repeatability of echocardiography outstrip any other pericardial effusion detecting technique.[56] Animal work confirmed the accuracy of this determination.

Detection of pericardial effusion was one of the first uses of echocardiography,[47] and for many laboratories and users it remains the major or only application of the technique. This is unfortunate, for the correct detection of pericardial effusion requires considerable skill and experience. It is difficult to imagine that one can have sufficient skill to recognize or negate the presence of pericardial effusion without interest or ability to image other cardiac structures. Therefore, we caution the user who "just wants to use echocardiography for detecting effusion."

Pericardial effusion is detected by passing a beam through the heart and into the lung. The effusion is recorded as a space, usually echo free, between the epicardium and the pericardium. It may appear anterior or posterior to the heart, or both.

In the normal echocardiogram, the pericardium is closely adherent to the epicardium, and, in fact, the two layers seldom can be resolved into separate structures. In patients with pericardial effusion, the two layers are separated by the effusion. Accordingly, identification of

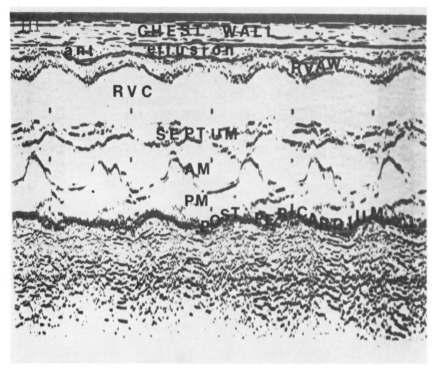

Fig. 4-35. — An example of a small anterior effusion, several hours post-operatively. Note that the pericardium probably is adherent to the right ventricular epicardium. This is particularly well seen just below the label *"ant."* The effusion probably is between the pericardium and the chest wall. No posterior pericardial effusion is present.

effusion requires positive identification of the anterior and posterior epicardium. It is necessary to record the endocardium as well as the epicardium to eliminate misidentification of effusion. Simultaneously recording the wall and the mitral valve as a marker of beam location is useful.

The posterior pleuropericardial interface usually can be found by decreasing the echograph gain control. This structure is the brightest trace in the posterior cardiac field, and in the normal usually is the last echo in that area to disappear as gain is decreased. However, some lung reflections may also be very bright. Identification of the posterior pericardium is slightly more difficult in the patient with an effusion because the echo is less intense than usual.

The anterior pericardium is more difficult to identify because the

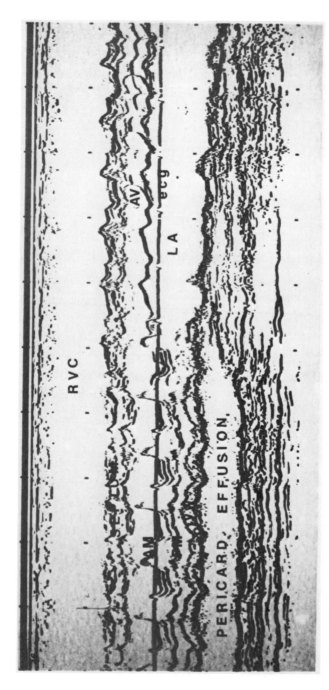

Fig. 4-36. – A large posterior pericardial effusion is seen behind the left ventricular epicardium. Note that the effusion ends at the junction of the left ventricle and left atrium. The right ventricular cavity is markedly dilated. This patient had a huge AV fistula and was in congestive failure at the time of this echocardiogram. This was a hemopericardium, etiology not known.

acoustic impedance mismatch between the chest wall and the pericardium is less than the mismatch between the air-filled lung and the pericardium. An anterior effusion is seen as a space between the chest wall and the anterior right ventricular wall. Occasionally, as shown in Figure 4-35, the effusion can be between the pericardium and the chest wall. The illustration was recorded postoperatively.

A posterior effusion is recorded as a space between the left ventricular epicardium and the pericardium. It is of considerable importance that pericardial effusions cannot form behind the left atrium because pulmonary veins bind the left atrial wall to the pericardial sac. Thus, the large effusion usually ends at the left ventriculo-left atrial junction (posteriorly) (Fig. 4-36). If an effusion is found behind the left atrium, it probably is pleural.[56] Occasionally, one can record

Fig. 4-37. — The space behind the left ventricular wall and the pericardium is a pseudo-effusion, and a phantom image is shown in the lung. It is evident that there is a thick, dense echo behind the posterior left ventricular wall, which is the pericardium. Phantom images can be quite troublesome and confusing. This patient had no cardiac disease.

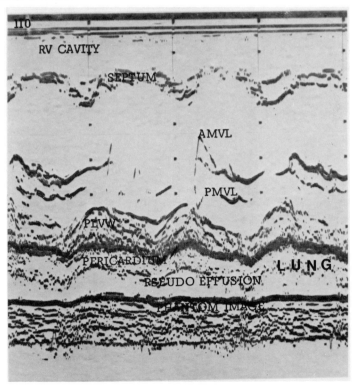

a combined pericardial and pleural effusion. In such an instance, the pericardium is recorded as the structure suspended between the two effusions. Further, left pleural effusions often are difficult to distinguish from pericardial effusions.

The echo-free space that represents the pericardial effusion occurs because there is no interface in the effusion. However, if the gain is turned too high, even the effusion can show echoes. Sometimes the posterior part of the effusion can present more than the expected number of echoes. This may be due to sedimentation of particles in the effusion. The examiner must use the echocardiograph skillfully to show the relatively echo-free area.

Phantom images can appear as dense lines behind the heart, and these can be confusing (Fig. 4-37). One differentiating feature between phantom images from the heart and the pericardial echo is that the latter has little, if any, motion when the effusion is present. However, lung reflections can also be stationary (Fig. 4-37).

The lung has a characteristic nondescript multiple reflecting appearance and usually looks somewhat stippled. This stippled-appearing lung fills in the concavity created by left ventricular contraction in the normal (Fig. 4-37). In patients with pericardial effusion, the lung does not fill in the space created by contraction of the heart but is separated from it by the effusion.

Accuracy in detecting effusions declines with the size of the effusion. Posterior systolic separation of epicardium and pericardium is relatively unimportant and was found in approximately half the individuals (adult) with less than 16 ml of effusion.[107] We found this sign in 10% of normal children. In adults, more than 16 ml of fluid caused diastolic and systolic separation.[107]

Systolic separation of the anterior right ventricular wall and chest wall (Fig. 4-38) is seen relatively commonly in normals and probably does not represent significant pathology.[56, 107] It may be due to the fact that we examine most subjects in the supine position. The right ventricular anterior wall does not necessarily adhere to the chest wall in this position, and contraction may pull the heart away from the anterior chest wall.

The size of the effusion is relatively easy to classify at both ends of the spectrum as very large or very small, but the exact volume has been difficult to estimate or compute.[174] In general, if an effusion is present anteriorly and posteriorly, it is relatively large. If the heart tends to "swing" with unusual motion in the effusion, the effusion probably is large. "Swinging" occurs as the result of excessive freedom of total cardiac motion in the fluid-filled pericardium. In this

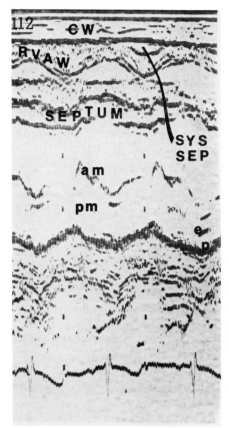

Fig. 4-38. — Pseudo-effusion. A systolic separation *(SYS SEP)* is seen anteriorly. The right ventricular anterior wall *(RVAW)* touches the chest wall *(CW)* during most of diastole. The anterior and posterior mitral valves *(am* and *pm)* are shown. The left ventricular wall is visible in the last beat to the right, and the endocardium *(e)* and pericardium *(p)* are marked.

state, the posterior-wall of the left ventricle and the septum move together and, at first glance, one might think that paradoxical septal motion is present. However, closer examination shows that this is an artifact of the "swinging heart." In fact, the heart may not return to its previous position with each beat. This lack of return may be registered on the electrocardiogram as electrical alternans.[56]

Our Experience with This Lesion:

Small pericardial effusions are far more common in patients with congenital cardiac disease than we suspected prior to examining by echocardiography. Effusions rather commonly accompany congestive cardiac failure and may accompany pneumonia.

Detection of effusion in the child is relatively easy if the examiner is experienced. This probably is because resolution of structures is easier to attain in the child than in the adult. On a few occasions, we have found unsuspected large effusions in patients who before the echocardiographic study were thought to have large hearts. The presence of a combined effusion (pericardial and pleural) can be diagnostically treacherous because one can misinterpret it as totally pericardial or totally pleural.

In one instance, we thought that we had made a significant error when no pericardial fluid could be withdrawn from a patient who had a classic-appearing pericardial effusion. At autopsy, the pericardium was filled with clotted blood. This was our only "false positive." This episode underscores the fact that echocardiography cannot suggest the type of fluid that will be found; it merely suggests that it is present.

Most tracings that we have seen that were erroneously diagnosed as pericardial effusion were prima facie evidence of poor technique.

Common errors include:

1. Mistaking a phantom image for the pericardium.

2. Mistaking the ventricular septum for the anterior right ventricular wall and the right ventricular cavity for an effusion.

3. Far medial angulations of the transducer show the right ventricular lateral wall and mediastinum. The latter can be mistaken for fluid (Fig. 4-39).

If a truly good study is obtained, misdiagnosis should be rare. However, not all studies can be excellent. For example, obtaining a very good study immediately postoperatively can be difficult. However, this is a time when pericardial effusion is a serious problem and the examiner must be most persistent.

Points of Caution:

1. Be certain to clearly identify the anterior and posterior cardiac walls and the pericardium. Simultaneous recording of the mitral leaflets is good practice.

2. Expect and recognize phantom images and lung reflections.

3. Although the first descriptions of pericardial effusion involve the use of A-mode, use of M-mode is preferable.

4. Alter the gain to clearly show the pericardium and rid the effusion of echoes.

5. Show the entire heart and chest wall on the recording.

6. Be certain that what is called a pericardial effusion stops at the left ventricular–left atrial junction. If it does not, observe layers carefully to rule out pleural effusion.

7. Avoid precise volume estimation. Estimates usually have been unsuccessful. Also, the effusion may be loculated.

8. Do not accuse the echocardiographic technique, which may

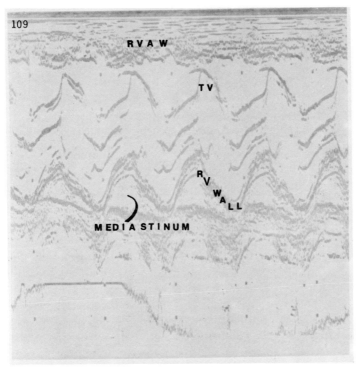

Fig. 4-39. — A pseudo-effusion can be demonstrated in normal individuals by tilting the transducer far to the right. The most distant moving part of the heart in this figure probably is the right ventricular wall. Mediastinal structures are adjacent to the right ventricular wall. This combination could be confused with posterior left ventricular wall and an effusion. The tricuspid valve *(TV)* and the right ventricular anterior wall *(RVAW)* are shown.

detect a very small effusion, of misdiagnosis if you cannot confirm the presence of the effusion by a less sensitive technique.

9. Far medial rotation of the transducer will show the tricuspid valve, right atrial or ventricular free wall and mediastinum. This can be confused with an effusion (Fig. 4-39).

5 / Examination of Patients

THE OBJECTIVE of echocardiographic examination of a patient is to obtain a high-quality diagnostic tracing. If this objective is accomplished, all other factors, such as control settings, selection of instruments and type of recording apparatus, become inconsequential. Unfortunately, performance of a proper echocardiogram is technically difficult and requires considerable experience and knowledge. Irrespective of prior training, a 3–6 month training period usually is required to get a consistently good examination. Additionally, continued exposure is necessary, for one gets out of practice quickly.

Conceptually, echocardiography differs from electrocardiography. The latter test is relatively easy to do. Within several hours, an intelligent technician can learn to obtain an electrocardiogram. The technician needs little interpretive knowledge to get a good study. The tracing can be read later by a physician. The opposite situation is true for an echocardiogram. While performing the examination, the echocardiographer must search for each structure, eliminate artifacts to the maximal extent possible and capture the true representation of the cardiac anatomy for hard copy. If an abnormality is present, he must recognize and record it in a manner that will be objective and convincing to others. Thus, the echocardiographer must recognize the abnormality. If the diagnosis is not recognized and thus not captured on paper, the likelihood is small that anyone could interpret the recording correctly at a later date. This fact accounts for the length of necessary training and the high pay of the echocardiographic technician.

If the number of echocardiograms performed in an institution is relatively large, a technician probably will be necessary unless the physician decides to devote his entire efforts to echocardiography. A single examination can take from 5 minutes to 1½ hours. For children, the average is about 10 minutes but for the adult it frequently is much longer. A technician can learn to perform and interpret echocardiography, but an interested and knowledgable physician working with the technician is mandatory for success. The physician must know more echocardiography, cardiac physiology and anatomy than the technician; otherwise, the technician will shoulder the burden of diagnosis alone.

GENERAL FEATURES OF THE EXAMINATION

For best results, the new echocardiographer should begin with a cooperative subject in order to achieve success. A sleeping child about 1 year of age is an excellent subject. Older individuals and those with emphysema are more difficult to study, and a few are impossible.

The examiner should sit comfortably on a chair of appropriate height to permit close observation of the echoscope. To free the hands, a foot pedal should be used to start the recorder or camera whenever a tracing is desired. We usually examine from the patient's left side, with the right hand holding the transducer, and use the left hand to control the echograph. A transducer should be selected that is of appropriate frequency and size for the objective of the study and the age of the individual. The examiner's arm should rest on the patient, the bed or some other structure. The heel of the hand and the fingers should rest on the chest to stabilize the transducer but still permit angulation (Fig. 5-1). Failure to rest the arm and hand will

Fig. 5-1.—This figure demonstrates the proper stabilization of a transducer. The first important aspect is to brace the fingers against the child's chest so that the transducer will be as stable as possible and move with the chest. The heel of the hand is rested on the child's shoulder and the examiner's elbow is on the mattress. This three-point stabilization provides maximal transducer control.

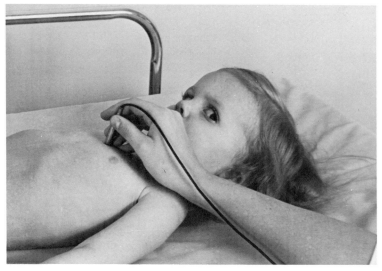

quickly result in fatigue and perhaps premature cessation of the examination. Under certain circumstances, the patient can be examined while he is sitting or even standing, but examiner arm fatigue is a limiting factor when the study is conducted in these positions.

An electrically controlled bed is useful for examining older children and adults. It is used to bring the patient to a 30–35° upright angle without the necessity for hand cranking or use of pillows. To observe certain structures, it is helpful to rotate the patient so that his left side is down.

An airless gel is used for coupling the transducer to the patient. We generally use Sonigel. This preparation does not stain clothing, and if it is not completely removed at the end of the examination, it will flake off as a white powder. On occasion, we have run out of the commercial preparation while doing echocardiograms in remote clinics and have used mineral oil, ECG electrode paste and antibiotic ointments with some success. At the end of the examination, the compound should be wiped from the transducer! Substitutes may be corrosive!

Distraction is in order for examination of the awake infant. A bottle of milk or sugar water may be the best distraction. Small children are examined more easily while being held by a parent. If the infant attempts to grab the transducer, try letting him hold an object in each hand. Securing the ECG leads to the child seems to be more traumatic than the remainder of the procedure, but we have found no simple solution to this problem. Fortunately, the echocardiographic examination of an infant takes only a few minutes, but these minutes frequently are filled with examiner and parental ingenuity, creativity and frustration. On occasion, we have resorted to sedation, but the need is rare. The persistent examiner usually is rewarded with an excellent study in the very young child.

THE TECHNIQUE

To begin the examination, one hand should hold the transducer and the other hand should be on the echographic controls. Initially, the transducer is placed in the fourth left interspace beside the sternum and held perpendicular to the chest wall. The "main bang" is positioned anteriorly, at the top of the oscilloscope. This prevents the frequent error of setting the anterior structures off the top of the oscilloscope. The total instrument gain is set at about three-fourths maximum. The unit then is switched to the A-mode and the depth adjusted to be appropriate for the age of the individual being studied. For the young child, we usually use about 4–5 cm in depth;

for the older child or adult, 10–12 cm is more appropriate. This is not a fixed rule, as hearts vary in size. While still on A-mode, the depth compensation is initially adjusted. A general suggestion is to start the slope at about half the depth and adjust the angle of the slope to be steep. The echograph then is switched to M-mode.

The first objective is to identify a landmark. If no obvious landmark is visible, look for an undulating motion and carefully and slowly change the angle of the transducer to the chest wall. Once an undulating motion or valve is sighted, "hone in" on the structure and alter the gain and reject controls to bring it clearly into view. The new examiner must "get the feel" of the transducer. The transducer angling technique involves making tiny, almost imperceptible, motions of the proximal portion of the transducer while not moving the distal portion (that portion in contact with the skin). These motions cause the beam angle to change with respect to the heart. The transducer can receive echoes only from structures that the beam strikes at the perpendicular. The reason that such small motions are required is that the chest wall acts as a fulcrum. A slight change in transducer angle sweeps a large section of the heart, as shown in Figure 5-2.

The anterior mitral valve leaflet usually is the structure to be located first. The anterior leaflet has one of the fastest excursions of any structure in the heart and is easily recognizable (Fig. 5-3). This leaflet serves as a landmark for other structures. Once the anterior leaflet

Fig. 5-2.—A transducer is pictured on the chest wall and the heart is anterior to the transducer. The chest wall acts as a fulcrum and very slight motion of the transducer will cause very large deviations of the beam in the more distant portions of the heart.

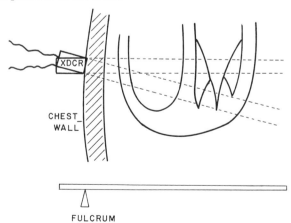

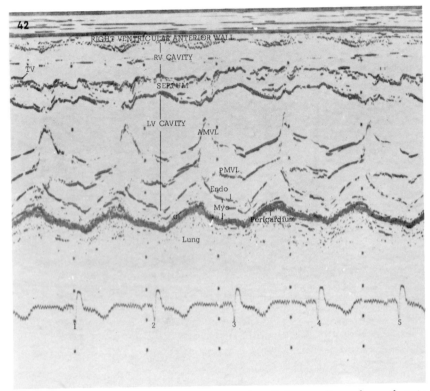

Fig. 5-3.—An echocardiographic example of the cardiac plane that is viewed when the beam passes through the posterior mitral leaflet. Abbreviations include: *RV* = right ventricle; *LV* = left ventricle; *AMVL* = anterior mitral valve leaflet; *PMVL* = posterior mitral valve leaflet; *Endo* = endocardium; *Myo* = myocardium; *TV* = tricuspid valve; *e* = epicardium. The portion of the tricuspid valve seen most likely is part of the chordae. Compare this echocardiogram with the diagram of the heart in Figure 5-4. Lines are used for cavity or wall identification, not for planes of measurement.

has been sighted, the controls should be used to resolve the valve to the extent possible. Enough rejection should be used to rid the cavity of extraneous echoes and gain should be adjusted to produce a clear image. At this point, we usually reset the slope to begin and end just in front of the septum or anterior tip of the anterior mitral leaflet or the anterior aortic wall.

The posterior leaflet of the mitral valve (Fig. 5-3) can be brought into view by tilting the transducer slightly leftward and inferiorly from the point where the anterior leaflet is found. Success in this maneuver is not always achieved easily. The posterior leaflet has a motion that is nearly a mirror image of the anterior mitral leaflet. If it cannot be found at this location, the examiner can try sliding the transducer slightly inferiorly or leftward.

The posterior leaflet of the mitral valve is a critical landmark, for when it is in view, numerous other structures can be viewed also. These structures include:

1. Anterior right ventricular wall.
2. Right ventricular cavity.
3. Ventricular septum.
4. The minor axis of the left ventricle.
5. The posterior left ventricular wall.
6. Occasionally the tricuspid valve.
7. Anterior and posterior pericardium.

Structures 1–5 are measured only when the posterior mitral valve is demonstrated. Comparison of Figure 5–3 with Figure 5–4 shows that most or all of the structures are perpendicular to the beam when it passes through the posterior mitral valve leaflet. Additionally, since the leaflet is small, the beam must be localized to the same position each time the valve is found. This improves measurement repeatability. The ideal echocardiogram of the area would show all structures simultaneously, but the ideal is not always achieved. Therefore, the objective becomes to demonstrate the structure(s) to the maximal extent possible while holding the posterior leaflet in view. Frequently, resolving one structure will hamper visualization of another. Several control settings and a few feet of paper may be required to see all structures with reference to the leaflet.

Fig. 5-4. — The heart is sectioned in the plane most often viewed by echocardiography, i.e., through the posterior mitral leaflet. See text for details.

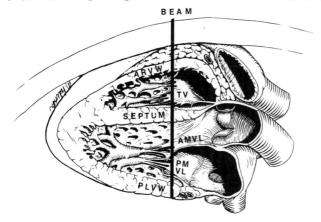

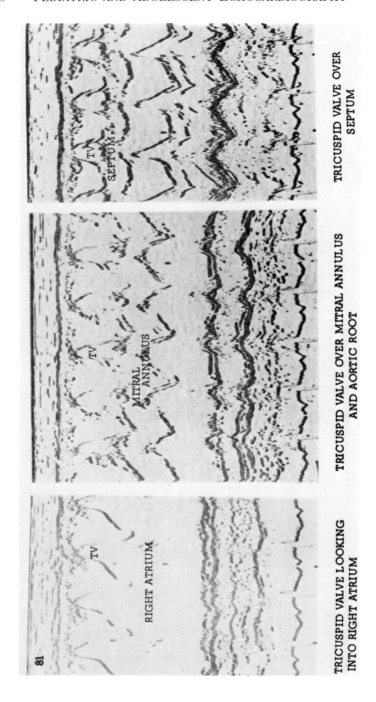

Fig. 5-5.—The tricuspid valve (*TV*) can be viewed from several angles. The left panel of this figure demonstrates the tricuspid valve as it appears when the transducer is pointing to the right lateral in the first frame. In this panel, the far structure is the right atrial wall. If the transducer is tilted slightly superiorly, the beam will pass through the tricuspid leaflet and also the mitral annulus (middle panel). If the beam is directed mainly posteriorly and slightly leftward, the tricuspid valve may be seen at the same time as the posterior mitral leaflet is viewed (right panel). In children, the tricuspid valve is observed most commonly in situations similar to the right-hand and left-hand panels and seen less commonly over the mitral annulus in normals.

The anterior wall of the right ventricle is difficult to record. If it is not visualized properly when the other structures are recorded, the following technique may be tried. First, use the highest-frequency transducer that will permit satisfactory penetration. Then, set the start of the depth compensation to begin in the middle of the right ventricular cavity. This permits the anterior right ventricular wall to be controlled solely with the near gain. Then adjust the near gain and reject very carefully to permit optimal visualization of this structure. In the adult and older child, use a high-frequency transducer to increase the chance for identification of this structure. The right ventricular wall should be recorded with simultaneous visualization of the posterior leaflet of the mitral valve so that orientation is preserved and a consistent area is evaluated.

The technical objective in studying the septum (Fig. 5-3) is to see discrete and complete right and left ventricular septal surfaces. The septum usually is recorded when the anterior and posterior leaflets are seen simultaneously. Often the septum appears to be broken. This is not usually evidence of a ventricular septal defect but is merely a result of beam angulation with respect to the septum. Again, minute readjustments of the angle are required to demonstrate this structure clearly. Leftward rotation of the patient may be helpful. In the difficult patient, slight anterior or posterior adjustment of the start of depth compensation may be useful.

The tricuspid valve (Fig. 5-5) has a motion similar to that of the mitral valve. One leaflet is attached to the septum. Sometimes it is visualized in front of the anterior aortic wall. It is a relatively easy structure to record in the child but is more difficult in the adult. In the child it frequently is visualized in the same plane that permits one to see both leaflets of the mitral valve, especially if the transducer is located medially. If it cannot be sighted from these positions, it frequently can be seen in excellent relief by angling the transducer rightward from the fourth left interspace in a plane nearly parallel with the anterior chest wall.

The posterior wall of the heart (Fig. 5-2) is best recorded in the same position that brings the posterior leaflet of the mitral valve into view. To start, find the combined echo of the epicardium and pericardium, which is a very bright line at the back of the heart. Little problem usually is encountered in identifying this structure. Occasionally, the structure is not as obvious as usual, and it can be sighted by decreasing the gain until only a single undulating line is seen at approximately the back of the heart. This line usually, but not always, is the epipericardium.

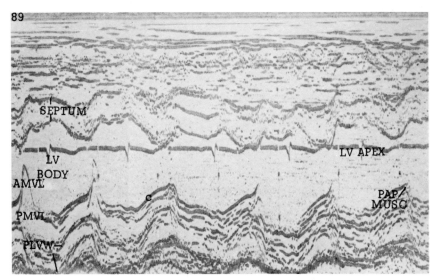

Fig. 5-6.—A sweep is demonstrated from the mitral valve to the papillary muscles. The papillary muscle demonstrates a much larger contraction than the posterior left ventricular wall. Chordae frequently are seen attaching the valve leaflet to the papillary muscle. *c* = chordae.

In the normal, the left ventricular endocardium has more motion than the pericardium and lies 1 cm or less anterior to it. In contrast to the pericardium, the endocardium is a thin structure, as the acoustic impedance mismatch between it and blood is less than that between the pericardium and the air-filled lung. Accordingly, the endocardium appears as a much thinner, fainter tracing. However, it is a very important structure to identify. Precise angulation and use of the damping control are helpful in identifying the endocardium.

After the posterior leaflet is sighted, the transducer should be tilted even more inferiorly, posteriorly and leftward in order to demonstrate the attachment of the leaflets to the chordae and the chordae to the papillary muscles (Fig. 5-6). A slight further angulation will bring the apex of the heart into view.

THE MITRAL TO AORTIC SWEEP

The transducer is angulated slowly anteriorly, rightward and superiorly from the point where the leaflets of the mitral valve are demonstrated so that it sweeps through an arc and ends up pointing toward the right shoulder. This motion should bring the aorta into

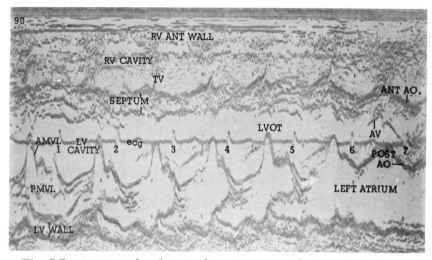

Fig. 5-7.—An example of a mitral aortic sweep. The important feature of this sweep is the demonstration of continuity of the mitral valve and the posterior aortic wall and the continuity of the septum and the anterior aortic wall.

Fig. 5-8.—An example of the aortic valve and left atrium. *RV* = right ventricle; *ANT AO WALL* = anterior aortic wall; *POST AO WALL* = posterior aortic wall; *AV* = aortic valve; *LA* = left atrium.

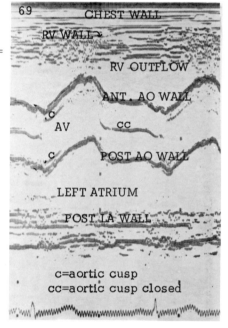

view. If the sweep is performed properly and the transducer is located over the anterior mitral valve ring, the anterior mitral valve leaflet will be seen to be continuous with the posterior wall of the aorta and the septum will blend into the anterior wall of the aorta (Fig. 5-7). If this sweep is performed from an unusual angle or very rapidly in the normal patient, these structures may seem to be discontinuous.

The aortic valve (Fig. 5-8) usually is visualized best within the aorta at a point in space just after the septum has blended into the anterior aortic wall and the mitral leaflet has formed the posterior aortic wall. Recording of the aortic valve in children is relatively easy, but in the adult it often requires more manipulation. Sometimes only one cusp can be seen at a time. Frequently, however, minute adjustments of the transducer or gain permit both cusps to come to view simultaneously.

The left atrium can be visualized as the space posterior to the aorta (Fig. 5-7). One technique for bringing out the aorta and the left atrium is to use the sloped depth compensation setting such that the slope begins at the anterior end of the heart and ends just behind the heart. This permits the near gain to control the entire echograph.

Fig. 5-9.—The pulmonary valve *(PV)* occasionally is viewed with an anterior and a posterior cusp as shown in this figure. Most commonly, the anterior cusp is not seen because it is parallel to the ultrasonic beam. The posterior cusp is observable in most patients. In contrast to the situation found in the aortic valve, multiple diastolic lines are rather common in the normal pulmonary valve.

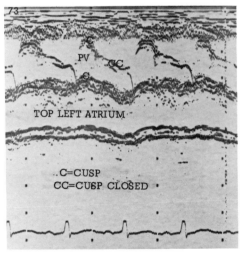

THE PULMONARY VALVE

The pulmonary valve is the most difficult of the four cardiac valves to identify and record (Fig. 5-9). Nonetheless, we are able to record it in almost all normal children. Several techniques are useful in searching for this structure. First, the pulmonary valve usually is visualized by moving the transducer one interspace cephalad to the point where the aortic valve is sighted. From this position, the transducer is angled slightly superiorly and laterally. If this does not bring the valve into view, the transducer may be positioned slightly more medially and then angled left lateral. If neither of these techniques works, the valve then can be sought in the general vicinity of the second or third interspace, 2–3 cm to the left of the sternum. Frequently, only the posterior cusp of the pulmonary valve is visualized. However, in infants two cusps commonly are seen. Inferior to the visualized cusp is a dense, thick echo, which represents the crista supraventricularis.

THE ELECTROCARDIOGRAM

The electrocardiogram is used as a reference tracing. Unfortunately, most instruments used today do not permit the tracing to be moved above the "main bang" and out of the way. Therefore, it must run through the cardiac echo and frequently it is lost in the myriad of echoes. There is no good place to put the electrocardiogram and it must be switched from one location to another.

THE SUPRASTERNAL APPROACH

The suprasternal approach is an uncomfortable, seldom used but important technique.[81] Figure 5-10 demonstrates that the beam from the suprasternal notch will pass through the arch of the aorta, the right pulmonary artery and the left atrium. Thus, two structures not usually evaluated and identified by echo can be studied and the left atrium can be measured in a second dimension (Fig. 5-11). Additionally, one can determine a right aortic arch by finding no aortic arch in the usual position but recording it with right angulation. The latter can be a particulary treacherous differential and requires considerable practice and experience.

We do a suprasternal study as part of our regular examination. It is performed by placing a small transducer in the suprasternal notch and angling it directly inferiorly. A small transducer is required to

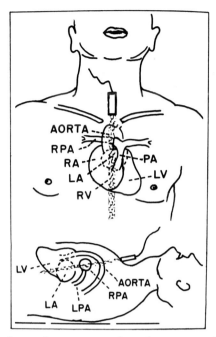

Fig. 5-10. — This figure demonstrates that a beam passed through the suprasternal notch will transect the aorta, the right pulmonary artery and the left atrium. This approach is very valuable for evaluating these structures and, in particular, the dimension of the left atrium in the Y coordinate. (Reproduced, with permission, from B. B. Goldberg.[81])

avoid inducing angulation by the larynx. The necessary depth setting is obvious from direct measurement of the chest.

The suprasternal examination usually is rather simple and all three structures are observed quickly. However, occasionally a patient is found in whom no structures can be sighted.

SUBXIPHOID APPROACH

Another somewhat unconventional approach described by Chang and Feigenbaum[22] is the subxiphoid approach. This was found to be useful in individuals with emphysema or lung covering the heart for another reason. It is performed by placing the transducer under the xiphoid and directing the beam superiorly and leftward. This is a very difficult approach but quite useful in individuals in whom no other approach is successful. Chang and Feigenbaum indicated that measurements obtained with this approach, with the exception of

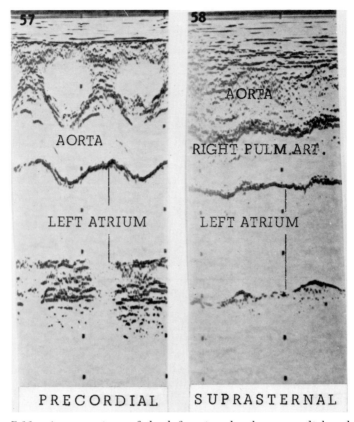

Fig. 5-11.—A comparison of the left atrium by the precordial and suprasternal approach. The left-hand panel demonstrates an example of the usual precordial approach. The aortic valve is within the aorta and the left atrium is measured at its widest point. The precordial measurement is 2.4 cm. From the suprasternal approach, the aorta, the right pulmonary artery and the left atrium are visualized. The superior border of the aorta is less clear than the inferior border. Left atrial dimension by this approach is 2.5 cm.

those of the right ventricle, are comparable to those obtained via the precordial approach. We have had only occasional experience with this technique, but it has considerable merit.

WARNING

Most of the errors that we have seen made and have made ourselves with echocardiography were the result of an inadequate study. Inadequate and subliminal information is worse than no information at all. It is possible to interpret nonbeautiful echocardiograms but it is not possible to interpret echocardiograms that do not have the necessary information. The echocardiographer must be willing to put forth the time and effort to do the job properly. If the examiner or equipment is not capable of performing the task, the task is better not performed. Normal and abnormal findings must be reproducible. The finding of one discontinuity or one unusual valve motion is not enough. Numerous recordings prove this point. We insist that the entire heart be on each recording. The isolation technique is not used, for we do not wish to risk disorientation. All structures must be seen in context with other structures. Do not attempt to save paper, as paper is far cheaper than errors. Every structure should be demonstrated and evaluated in every examination. This compulsiveness may seem overstressed, but in final evaluation it is not.

NOTES

6 / Self-Assessment Single Crystal Echocardiography

IN THIS CHAPTER we will present fragments of echocardiograms that are useful for provoking frustration, discussion, concentration and disagreement. Interpreting someone else's complete echocardiogram is difficult; interpreting someone else's fragments approaches impossibility. The tracings presented in Chapter 6 are intended to present classic examples, pitfalls in diagnosis and technique, and examples of difficulty in applying published criteria. A superficial approach to the example will bring all of our cautions and warnings to light. A systematic search of the echocardiogram for artifact, qualitative data and quantitative data from each beat will yield the best results. For maximal instruction:

1. Commit yourself by writing your answers before turning to the answer page.

2. Comment on each structure.

3. Quantitate every measurable structure and compare that measurement to the normal.

4. Do not totally reject any echo as totally inadequate (not all children are angels while being studied).

5. If your assessment disagrees with ours, you may be correct.

In preparing the problems for this chapter, the authors circulated echocardiographic fragments among themselves and others and found it a very cathartic experience (*Webster's Dictionary* defines cathartic as "elimination of a complex by bringing it to consciousness and affording it expression").

Enjoy!

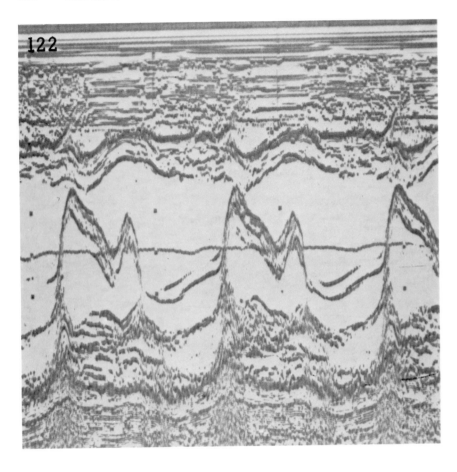

PROBLEM 1

This child had a body surface area of 1.58 m².

Reader's interpretation: _____

_____

_____

Measurements: _____

_____

_____

Diagnosis: _____

_____

_____

The most striking feature of this echocardiogram is the posterior systolic motion of the mitral leaflets, beginning with systole. In the normal, the closed leaflets should move anteriorly with systole. Mitral systole begins at the echocardiographic C point. With mitral prolapse, the posterior motion frequently begins later in systole than is shown in this example. In those instances, anterior motion would begin at C, but motion of one or both leaflets would reverse at approximately midsystole.

Other Features of This Echocardiogram:

1. The mitral diastolic tracing shows some low-amplitude, high-frequency vibration. If coarse low-frequency vibration or high-amplitude, high-frequency vibrations were present, aortic insufficiency would have to be considered. Low-amplitude, high-frequency vibrations commonly occur in normals and abnormals.

2. The double anterior mitral valve leaflet lines probably are not significant. These can occur in normals or abnormals. In posterior prolapse, the leaflets may contain excessive tissue, and multiple surfaces are more likely to be subtended by the beam. However, echo duplications of the valve should not be considered a diagnostic feature, for they can be seen in normals also.

3. The structure posterior to the mitral valve leaflet is the junction of the posterior left ventricular wall and left atrial wall. Part of the prolapse may extend into this area.

4. Septal motion is normal.

5. Note the recording of a small part of the tricuspid leaflet.

Criticisms of This Echocardiogram:

1. The anterior right ventricular wall is not seen.

2. The electrocardiogram is visible but the QRS is partially hidden by the anterior mitral valve leaflet.

3. A clearer posterior wall definition is desirable.

Pertinent Measurements:

1. Septal thickness is 0.6 cm.

2. E – F mitral slope is 102 mm/sec.

3. Posterior left ventricular wall, left ventricular internal dimension and right ventricular wall are not measurable.

Clinical Comment:

This patient had an apical early systolic click followed by a murmur. It became holosystolic when she sat up, and we recorded the echocardiogram in that position. She also had a hypoplastic right thorax. At catheterization, her mitral prolapse was marked. Repair of the chest wall did not improve the findings of prolapse. Mitral prolapse is common in patients with pectus excavatum and chest wall

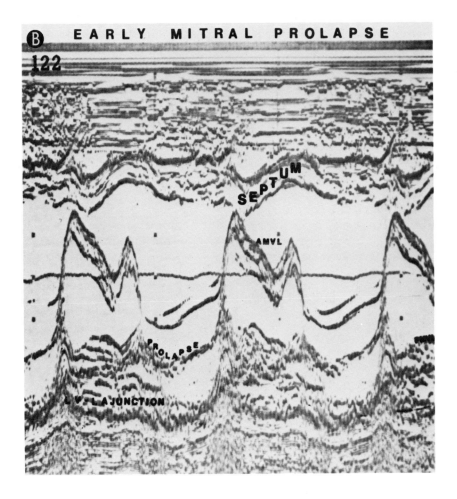

deformity. It now is clear that many of the "unusual murmurs" in these patients are due to mitral prolapse.

Pertinent literature references: see Chapter 4, Section 4.13.

NOTES

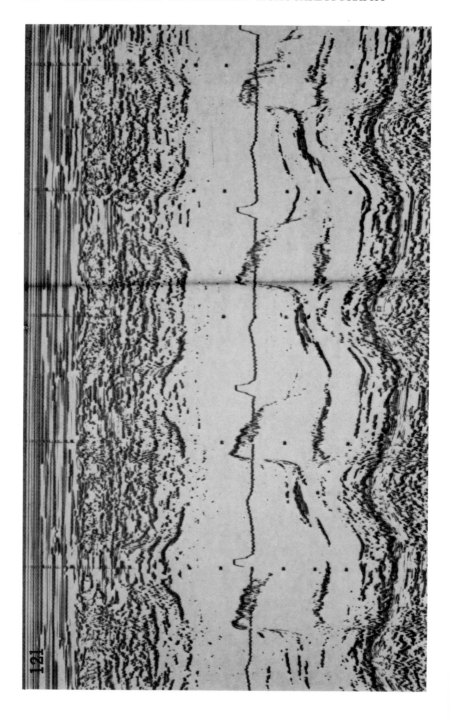

PROBLEM 2

This child had a body surface area of 1.71 m².

Reader's interpretation: _____

_____

_____

Measurements: _____

_____

_____

Diagnosis: _____

_____

_____

_____

The most striking feature of this echocardiogram is the coarse diastolic vibration of the anterior mitral valve leaflet. This is particularly well demonstrated in diastole of beat 1. Coarse vibration at the anterior mitral leaflet is created by the interplay of two forces:

1. Flow of blood through the mitral valve from the left atrium.
2. Flow of blood back into the outflow tract of the left ventricle as the result of aortic insufficiency.

The E–F slope of the first three complexes is 97 mm/sec. Merely visualizing the slope would suggest mitral stenosis. However, measurement of this slope indicates that it is normal. The appearance probably is due to the high end diastolic pressure in the left ventricle. The patient does not have mitral stenosis. One can be reasonably certain of this from the echocardiogram by noting the normal motion of the posterior mitral leaflet.

Other Features of This Echocardiogram:
Posterior left ventricular wall and septum are 0.85 cm thick. An occasional normal of 1.7 m² will reach this thickness, but such thickness is on the very edge of the normal range. The left ventricular posterior wall is seen clearly and can be measured in all beats. The right ventricular side of the septum is less clear but can be measured in beat 2.

It might be suggested that very slight mitral systolic anterior motion might be present, but it is doubtful. Note this to be parallel to posterior heart wall motion, probably reflecting anterior motion of the entire heart.

The Vcf equals 0.45 circumferences/sec. This is reduced despite a volume overload. The reduction may suggest poor muscle function.

Criticisms of This Echocardiogram:
1. The right ventricular anterior wall is not visualized clearly, and it definitely should be studied in a patient with aortic insufficiency. It probably could have been recorded better if the depth compensation had been set near the septum and the anterior gain had been reduced. Switching to a higher-frequency transducer for this phase of the examination often is useful.
2. Better visualization of the mitral valve during systole would be desirable.

Pertinent Measurements:
1. Left ventricular posterior wall and septum = 0.85 cm.
2. Left ventricular internal dimension (diastolic) = 6.2 cm (> 95%) and left ventricular internal dimension (systolic) = 5 cm (> 95%).
3. Mitral E–F slope = 97 mm/sec.
4. Systolic time determined by the mitral valve = 0.43 sec.
5. Vcf = 0.45 circumferences/sec (abnormally low).

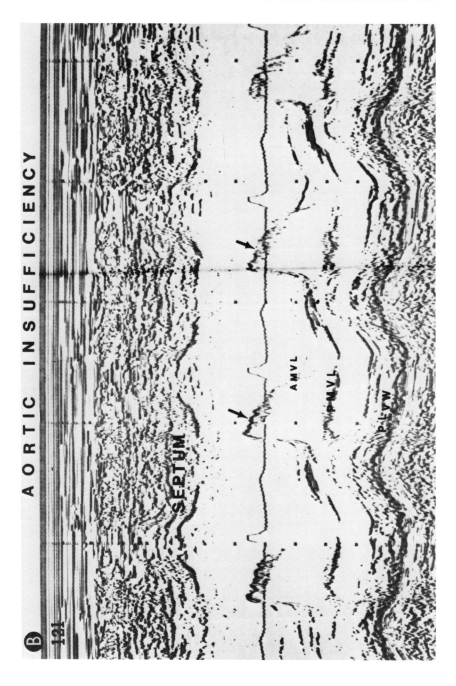

Clinical Comment:

It is not surprising that the left ventricular posterior wall and septum are hypertrophied or that the $LVID_s$ and $LVID_d$ are enlarged in this 13-year-old patient with isolated severe rheumatic aortic insufficiency. The Vcf is low, and this suggests that compensation is incomplete.

Pertinent literature references: see Chapter 4, Section 4.8.

NOTES

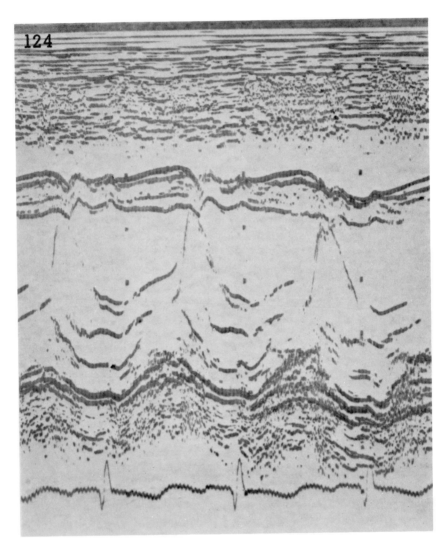

PROBLEM 3

This child had a body surface area of 0.7 m².

Reader's interpretation: _____

_____

_____

Measurements: _____

_____

_____

Diagnosis: _____

_____

_____

_____

The only significant abnormality in this tracing is the flat septal motion. Following the QRS, there is a very slight posterior motion followed by a flat left ventricular septal surface motion. It can be seen that the right ventricular septal surface moves anteriorly during systole, thus constricting the right ventricular cavity. This motion is paradoxical, Type B.

The right ventricular cavity appears to be somewhat enlarged, but its exact dimension is not known. It is at least 1.25 cm (beat 3) but may be larger.

Other Features of This Echocardiogram:

1. The posterior left ventricular wall is exaggerated and moves anteriorly 1 cm. This commonly occurs when the left ventricular posterior wall must make up for inadequate function of another portion of the left ventricle.

2. The epicardium and pericardium are continuously separated. This is visualized best in a portion of the echo preceding and following beat 1. This probably is evidence of a small effusion.

Criticism of This Echocardiogram:

The most serious criticism of this study is failure to demonstrate the anterior right ventricular wall.

Pertinent Measurements:

1. Left ventricular posterior wall = 0.4 cm.
2. Septum = 0.47 cm.
3. Left ventricular internal dimension (diastolic) = 2.9 cm (< 5%).
4. Mitral valve systolic time = 0.24 sec.
5. Vcf = 1.44 circumferences/sec. The significance of this measurement in view of paradoxical septal motion is not known.

Clinical Comment:

The echocardiogram was obtained immediately postoperatively on a patient who had repair of an atrial secundum defect. Preoperatively, he had paradoxical septal motion of the Type A variety, but postoperatively it changed to Type B. This probably indicates that the hinge point of the septum shifted superiorly following relief from the volume overload. The right ventricular cavity was larger preoperatively.

The echo is normal 1 year later. The measurements show that the $LVID_d$ is abnormally small. This is not unusual in patients with secundum defects. Frequently, the aortic dimension is also below the fifth percentile. Note that the $LVID_s$ was not measured. In the patient with paradoxical septal motion, the significance of this measurement is not clear.

Pertinent literature references: see Chapter 4, Section 4.1.

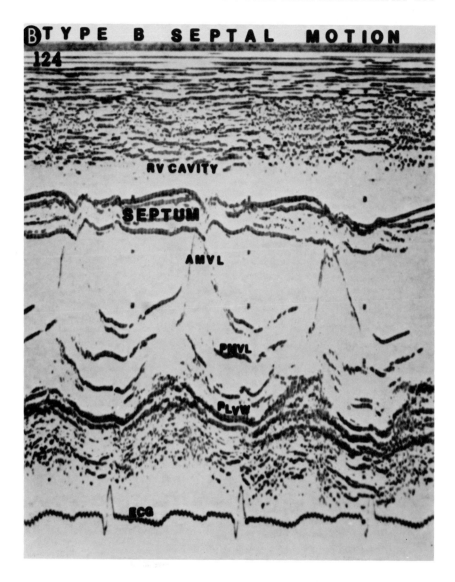

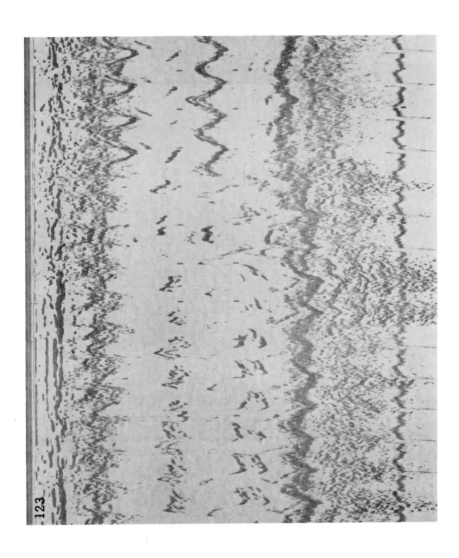

PROBLEM 4

This child had a body surface area of 0.3 m².

Reader's interpretation: _____

_____

_____

Measurements: _____

_____

_____

Diagnosis: _____

_____

_____

_____

A quick perusal of this echocardiogram may be misleading. First, it appears to be a low-quality tracing with little information. However, closer examination is required. Clearly, it is the tracing of an infant, because the cardiac depth is only 4.5 cm. However, the aorta is large by comparison with the left atrium and is beyond the ninety-fifth percentile for age. The measurements are 1.6 and 1.4 cm, respectively. The anterior aortic wall does not align with the septum, but overrides it anteriorly by 6 mm in diastole. Thus, septal aortic continuity is not present, and this finding suggests the diagnosis of tetralogy of Fallot. The posterior aortic wall is not clearly attached to the mitral valve. Certainly the systolic depth of the posterior aorta and the mitral valve are different. Could this represent a double outlet right ventricle? It is our opinion that the presence or absence of mitral-aortic continuity is difficult to judge. There is a suggestion of continuity in the beat preceding the first visualization of the posterior aortic wall. Other tracings from this patient clearly demonstrated mitral aortic continuity.

The septum appears broken and poorly recorded. This probably is because the beam was directed high, through the ventricular septal defect, and only occasionally caught the edge of the septum.

Occasionally, one can become confused by the similar level of the aortic valve closure line and the septum in tetralogy of Fallot or truncus arteriosus. If the systolic closure line is confused with the anterior aortic wall, "continuity" frequently will appear to be present.

Other Features of This Echocardiogram:

1. The right ventricular anterior wall is thickened beyond twice normal (0.65 cm). This is measured best in beat 4.

2. The mitral valve appears normal.

Criticism of This Echocardiogram:

Obviously, this tracing was not selected as an outstanding example of technique, yet it shows the features of tetralogy of Fallot. It would have been technically more perfect if the mitral aortic continuity were demonstrated and if the right ventricular anterior wall were delineated more precisely. It is doubtful if the septum could be recorded better at this level, because it is not intact.

Pertinent Measurements:

1. Aorta = 1.6 cm ($>95\%$).

2. Left atrium = 1.4 cm ($<5\%$).

3. Aortic valve opening = 1.15 cm (measurement at the last beat) ($>95\%$).

4. Right ventricular anterior wall = 0.65 cm ($>95\%$).

5. Left ventricular cavity is too poorly seen to measure.

6. Left ventricular posterior wall = 0.3 cm ($<5\%$).

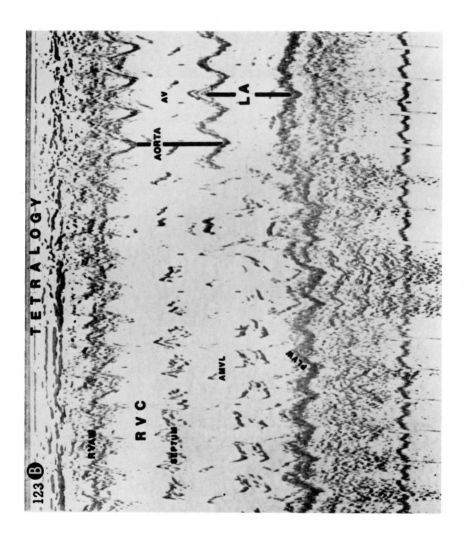

Clinical Comment:

Obviously, this infant has tetralogy of Fallot. Classic hallmarks are present in the measurements as well as in the qualitative aspects. The aortic dimension and valve separation are in excess of the ninety-fifth percentile. Aortic override is present. Right ventricular hypertrophy is present. The left atrium is small (< 5%) because of decreased lung blood flow. The left ventricular posterior wall is less than the fifth percentile in thickness.

Pertinent literature references: see Chapter 4, Section 4.21.

NOTES

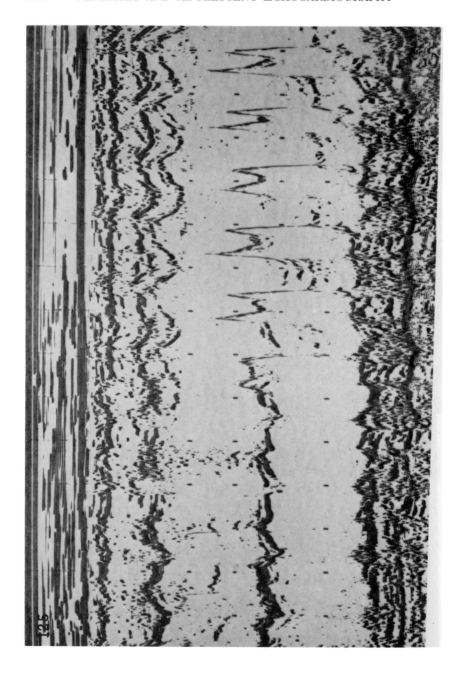

PROBLEM 5

This child had a body surface area of 0.9 m².

Reader's interpretation: _____

_____

_____

Measurements: _____

_____

_____

Diagnosis: _____

_____

_____

_____

The most unique features of this echocardiogram include the large aorta (2.6 cm) compared with the smaller left atrium (2.0 cm). This aortic root size is reminiscent of that seen in tetralogy of Fallot or truncus arteriosus. Poststenotic dilatation observed in aortic stenosis is different because it usually occurs higher in the aorta. It is of interest that the right ventricular dimension and the width of the right ventricular outflow tract are very narrow. Mitral configuration is unusual because of the tall A waves, which suggest a high end diastolic left ventricular pressure. Septal motion is normal. The left ventricle is dilated. Although not clearly delineated, a small pericardial effusion is present behind the left ventricular posterior wall, seen in both systole and diastole (last beat). This probably is due to the fact that the patient was in congestive failure.

Other Features of This Echocardiogram:
1. No tricuspid valve is seen, but this does not prove its absence. The area recorded is not the best for finding the tricuspid leaflet.
2. Septal motion is normal.

Criticism of This Echocardiogram:
The effusion is not convincing in this view. More rejection and less gain probably would have improved the appearance of the effusion and the right ventricular cavity (and eliminated the aortic valve cusp, as well). The posterior left ventricular wall is not clear. The electrocardiogram is imperceptibly buried in the lung.

Pertinent Measurements:
1. Aortic root = 2.6 cm (> 95%).
2. Aortic cusp opening = 1.6 cm (> 95%).
3. Left atrial dimension = 2.3 cm (< 5%).
4. Left ventricular posterior wall = 0.6 cm (> 95%).
5. Right ventricular anterior wall = 0.35 cm (> 95%).
6. Septal thickness = 0.5 cm (< 5%).
7. Left ventricular internal dimension (diastolic) = 4.75 cm (> 95%).
8. Left ventricular internal dimension (systolic) = 3.8 cm (> 95%).
9. Systolic time = 0.35 sec.
10. Vcf = 0.57 circumferences/sec (depressed).

Clinical Comment:
This 8-year-old boy had tricuspid atresia with a right Glenn and a left Blalock. The aortic root, valve separation and all left ventricular measurements exceed the ninety-fifth percentile. The left atrium is small because the shunts are relatively small and pulmonary blood flow is low. The right ventricular anterior wall in the outflow tract probably is thickened because of the pulmonary stenosis. These

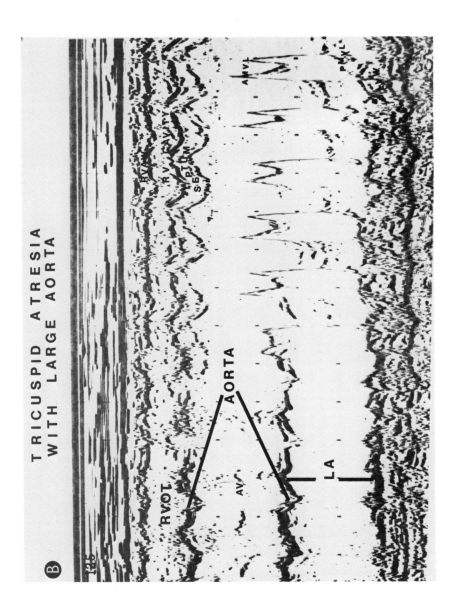

findings are in general accord with known pathology in this condition.

Pertinent literature references: see Chapter 4, Section 4.18.

NOTES

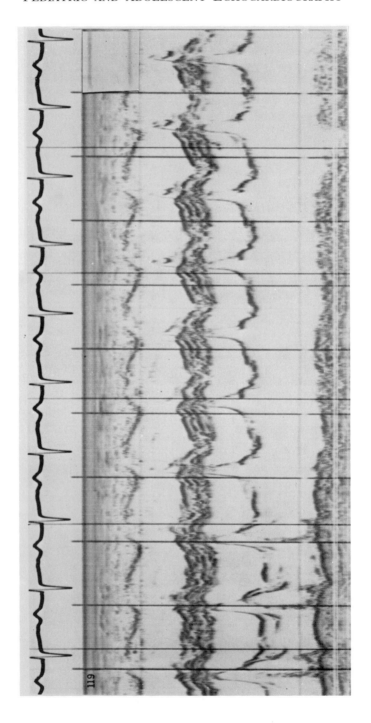

PROBLEM 6

This child had a body surface area of 0.3 m².

Reader's interpretation: _____

_____

_____

Measurements: _____

_____

_____

Diagnosis: _____

_____

_____

_____

This is an interesting sweep from the area that appears to be a mitral valve toward, but not into, the aorta. A number of findings are evident:

1. Posterior to the structure that appears to be the anterior and posterior leaflet of the mitral valve is the left atrial wall rather than the left ventricular wall.

2. The atrioventricular valve clearly bites into, and appears to go through, the septum.

3. The right ventricular anterior wall is excessively thick (0.6 cm).

4. Septal motion is normal in the plane of the posterior mitral leaflet.

5. The structure that appears to be the mitral valve is distorted.

6. Two different leaflet structures appear to move anteriorly in the diastole of, and before, beat 1.

These findings are common in patients with complete atrioventricular canals. The mitral valve is in a different plane than usual, accounting for the lack of left ventricular posterior wall below the valve. Septal thickness (0.6 cm) possibly is related to the right ventricular hypertrophy. The atrioventricular valve in this patient was a very primitive one, consisting of two common atrioventricular leaflets that passed through the septum. Exactly which portion of the leaflet is viewed in this particular echocardiogram is not certain.

Criticisms of This Echocardiogram:

1. The chest wall is not clearly separated from the right ventricle.

2. It would have been instructive to show a sweep from the papillary muscle to the aorta, but this was too long to photograph. The mitral to aortic sweep is difficult in the distorted anatomy of endocardial cushion defect patients. It should be noted that this particular sweep took only 5.2 seconds to accomplish.

3. Extraneous time lines are present.

Pertinent Measurements:

1. Right ventricular anterior wall = 0.6 cm (> 95%).

2. Septum = 0.6 cm (> 95%).

Clinical Comment:

This patient was a mongoloid child who had a complete canal.

The ventricular septal thickness is quite common in children with canal defects, and the reason is not clear. No left ventricular measurements were possible because the mitral valve was displaced, and the chamber posterior to the valve is the left atrium.

In view of the pulmonary vascular obstructive disease that the child exhibited at catheterization, the thickened right ventricular wall is to have been expected.

Pertinent literature references: see Chapter 4, Section 4.5.

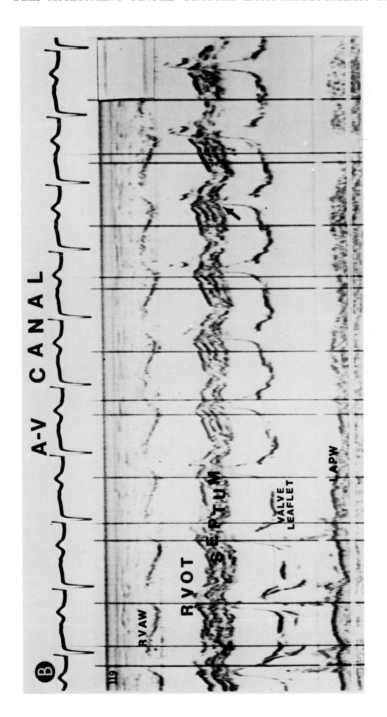

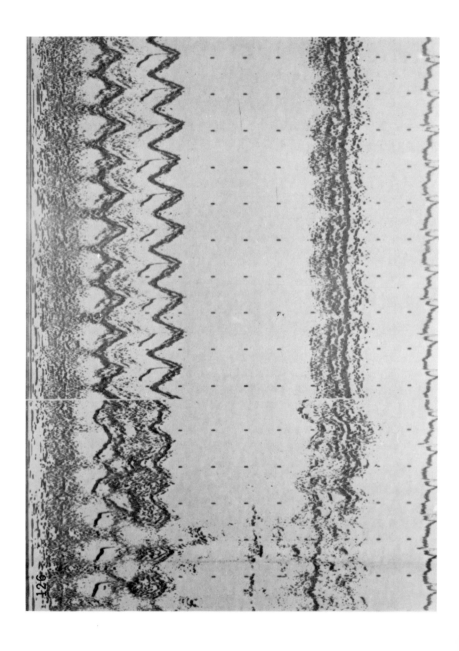

PROBLEM 7

This child had a body surface area of 0.55 m².

Reader's interpretation: _____

_____

_____

Measurements: _____

_____

_____

Diagnosis: _____

_____

_____

_____

The most obvious feature of this study is the huge size of the left atrium—approximately 5.6 cm. The aorta is much smaller—1.7 cm. The aortic valve appears normal. The left atrium is enlarged because of mitral insufficiency. The exact posterior margin of the left atrium is difficult to determine in this picture but probably is line 1 or line 2.

The section to the left was recorded only an instant before and shows the pulmonary valve and the crista supraventricularis.

Criticism of This Echocardiogram:
The posterior left atrial wall is indistinct.

Pertinent Measurements:
1. Left atrium = 5.6 cm (> 95%).
2. Aorta = 1.8 cm (> 95%).
3. Aortic cusp separation = 1.2 cm (> 95%).

Clinical Comment:
This 4-year-old child had rheumatic mitral disease and then a severe recurrence when she did not receive her prophylactic penicillin. At the time of this echocardiogram, she had clinical pulmonary edema. It is not at all surprising that her left atrium was massively dilated. Her last examination, 6 months after this study, showed a left atrium of 2.9 cm. We do not know why her aorta is enlarged. No aortic valve disease is obvious by examination. She has not been catheterized.

Pertinent literature references: see Chapter 4, Section 4.12.

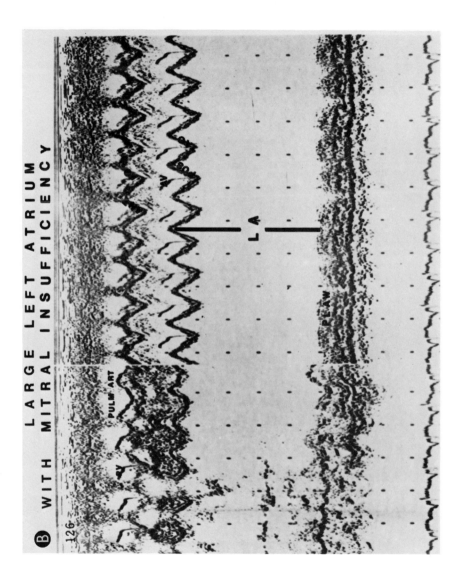

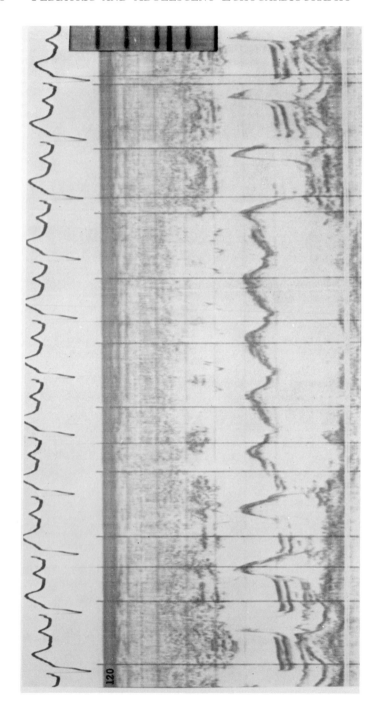

PROBLEM 8

This child had a body surface area of 0.36 m².

Reader's interpretation: _____

_____

_____

Measurements: _____

_____

_____

Diagnosis: _____

_____

_____

This echocardiogram demonstrates the complexity of interpreting relationships and structures with single crystal echocardiography. A continuous sweep from the mitral valve to a great vessel and back to the mitral valve is shown in a patient with autopsy-proved double outlet right ventricle. Either type of continuity or discontinuity that one wishes to describe is present. On the right, the anterior mitral valve leaflet seems to be discontinuous with the great vessel. The systolic level of the valve and the posterior great vessel wall are clearly dissimilar. On the left side of the strip, a totally different type of relationship is seen. The great vessel is clearly "continuous" with the anterior mitral valve leaflet.

The line between beats 7 and 8 is a paper fold and not a splice. The posterior mitral valve leaflet and posterior left ventricular wall are clearly visualized on both sides. The structure behind the great vessel is the left atrium

The great vessel walls are not visualized simultaneously. This occurs because the posterior wall is at a different level than the anterior, i.e., the great vessel is tilted with respect to the echo beam. Such a tilt commonly is seen during a sweep in patients with double outlet right ventricle, some transpositions and some truncus arterioses. It should be recalled that the normal aorta is also tilted slightly but less so. In normals, the angle of the beam, which is moving from the mitral valve to the aorta, usually bisects both walls of the aorta simultaneously, or nearly simultaneously. The point of this figure is to demonstrate the difficulty in evaluating mitral continuity with a single crystal echocardiographic instrument.

Criticism of This Echocardiogram:

The septum is visualized only in beats 2, 3 and 10, and questionably visualized in beat 9.

Pertinent Measurements:

1. Left atrium = 3.3 cm (> 95%) if it can be measured in this plane, and we are not certain that it can be. The great vessel valve is not visualized.

2. Left ventricular posterior wall = 0.5 cm.

3. Mitral valve E – F slope = 115 mm/sec.

Clinical Comment:

This child had a double outlet right ventricle with the aorta related to the ventricular septal defect. The mitral ring was closely related to the aortic ring. Only the edge of the defect separated the two.

It is not surprising that the left atrium was enlarged, for pulmonary blood flow was excessive. The ventricular septal defect was not ob-

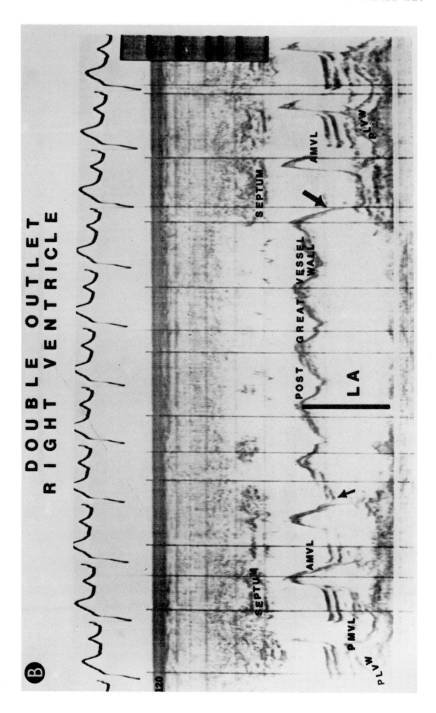

structive, and this may account for the lack of left ventricular hypertrophy.

Pertinent literature references: see Chapter 4, Section 4.23.

NOTES

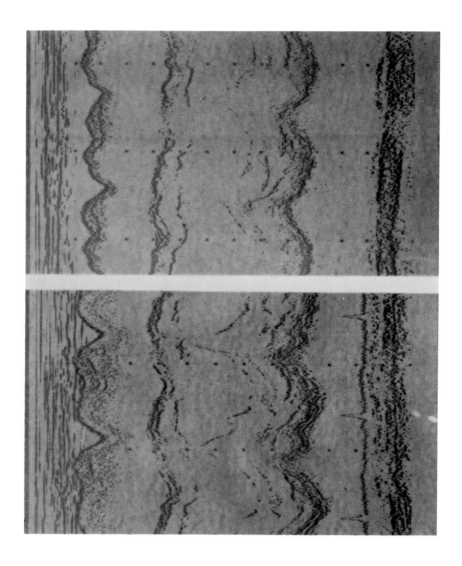

PROBLEM 9

This is an echocardiogram of a 12-year-old girl with a body surface area of 1.6 m². The left panel was taken with the patient supine and the right panel is the echocardiogram with the patient sitting.

Reader's interpretation: ⎯⎯⎯⎯⎯⎯⎯⎯⎯⎯⎯⎯⎯⎯⎯⎯

⎯⎯⎯⎯⎯⎯⎯⎯⎯⎯⎯⎯⎯⎯⎯⎯⎯⎯⎯⎯⎯⎯⎯⎯⎯⎯⎯⎯⎯

⎯⎯⎯⎯⎯⎯⎯⎯⎯⎯⎯⎯⎯⎯⎯⎯⎯⎯⎯⎯⎯⎯⎯⎯⎯⎯⎯⎯⎯

Measurements: ⎯⎯⎯⎯⎯⎯⎯⎯⎯⎯⎯⎯⎯⎯⎯⎯⎯⎯⎯⎯⎯

⎯⎯⎯⎯⎯⎯⎯⎯⎯⎯⎯⎯⎯⎯⎯⎯⎯⎯⎯⎯⎯⎯⎯⎯⎯⎯⎯⎯⎯

⎯⎯⎯⎯⎯⎯⎯⎯⎯⎯⎯⎯⎯⎯⎯⎯⎯⎯⎯⎯⎯⎯⎯⎯⎯⎯⎯⎯⎯

Diagnosis: ⎯⎯⎯⎯⎯⎯⎯⎯⎯⎯⎯⎯⎯⎯⎯⎯⎯⎯⎯⎯⎯⎯⎯

⎯⎯⎯⎯⎯⎯⎯⎯⎯⎯⎯⎯⎯⎯⎯⎯⎯⎯⎯⎯⎯⎯⎯⎯⎯⎯⎯⎯⎯

⎯⎯⎯⎯⎯⎯⎯⎯⎯⎯⎯⎯⎯⎯⎯⎯⎯⎯⎯⎯⎯⎯⎯⎯⎯⎯⎯⎯⎯

⎯⎯⎯⎯⎯⎯⎯⎯⎯⎯⎯⎯⎯⎯⎯⎯⎯⎯⎯⎯⎯⎯⎯⎯⎯⎯⎯⎯⎯

The diagnosis in this case is pericardial effusion. A 2.5-cm posterior epipericardial separation (supine) and a 3.3-cm separation (sitting) is present. An anterior epipericardial separation is also present and is greatest with the patient sitting.

The patient presented with a 2-week history of malaise, cough and shortness of breath. The echocardiogram was done on arrival and a diagnosis was reached. Taking the echocardiogram in sequence, note that just below the chest wall, the right ventricular anterior wall is quite contractile and is separated from the chest wall. This is especially notable while the patient is sitting. The echo is in the plane of the posterior mitral valve leaflet. The right ventricular cavity is slightly dilated. The motion of the interventricular septum is rather flat. The left ventricular posterior wall contracts normally after the QRS complex, but the electrocardiogram is missing in the right panel. This is a technical error. A pericardial tap produced clinical improvement, and "cardiomegaly" on chest roentgenograms disappeared. The effusion did not recur.

Criticisms of This Echocardiogram:

Technical errors in these echoes include:

1. No visible electrocardiogram in the right panel of the echocardiogram. The electrocardiogram is lost in the lung field. This is a constant problem with certain echographs.

2. The right ventricular anterior wall echo in the first echocardiogram is not clear. After beat 2, a discretely thin wall is observable. This thickness can be compared with that in the right-hand panel echo, which is clearer, confirming measurement of the right ventricular anterior wall.

3. A left ventricular to aortic sweep is not shown, but was performed. The sweep is useful, as the effusion almost invariably stops at the left ventricular posterior wall – left atrial junction.

Pertinent Measurements:

	SUPINE	SITTING
1. Right ventricular anterior wall	0.23 cm	0.23 cm
2. Right ventricular cavity	2 cm (> 95%)	2–3 cm (respiratory variation, see Chapter 3)
3. Septum (do not confuse tricuspid echoes above the septum with septal echoes)	0.73 cm (> 95%)	0.73 cm

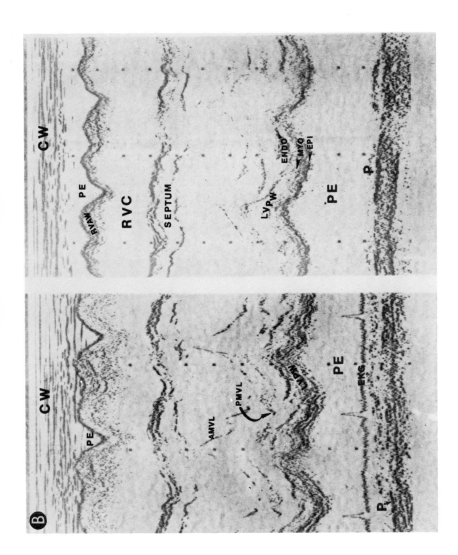

4. Left ventricular end
   diastolic dimension   4.0 cm (< 5%)   4.0 – 4.2 cm
5. Left ventricular posterior
   wall   0.75 cm   0.75 cm
6. Epipericardial sepa-
   ration (heavy line is
   pericardium, fine lines
   are artifact)
      Anterior   0.6 cm   1.6 cm
      Posterior   2.5 cm   3.3 cm
7. Vcf   1.00 circumfer-
                                ences/sec

Clinical Comment:

The left ventricular end diastolic dimension is less than the fifth percentile. The right ventricular cavity is greater than the ninety-fifth percentile. This might imply that the effusion changed cardiac geometry. Lack of right ventricular hypertrophy indicates lack of chronically elevated pulmonary vascular pressure. The septal measurement of greater than the ninety-fifth percentile is not explained.

Pertinent literature references: see Chapter 4, Section 4.33.

NOTES

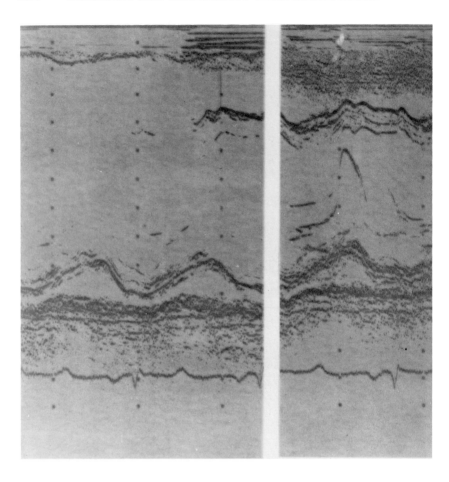

PROBLEM 10

This is an echocardiogram performed on a 12-year-old girl with a body surface area of 1.6 m².

Reader's interpretation: _____

_____

_____

Measurements: _____

_____

_____

Diagnosis: _____

_____

_____

_____

You guessed it! This echo is normal. This is the postpericardial tap echocardiogram taken on the patient described in echo Problem 9. The left panel of the echocardiogram shows the effect of changing gain settings to elucidate the right ventricular anterior wall. As the gain is increased, the right ventricular anterior wall clarity is lost, septal echoes are noted and it is seen that the echocardiogram is in the plane of the posterior mitral valve leaflet. The echogram at the right was performed using even more gain. Now, more discrete mitral valvular structures are noted and more definition is given to the septum and the posterior structures. Note that there no longer is significant epipericardial separation and the echogram is normal. Technically, this is a better echocardiogram in that the electrocardiogram is seen on both tracings.

Criticism of This Echocardiogram:

Septal and left ventricular posterior wall measurements could be confusing, as chordae are overlying the left ventricular posterior wall and the tricuspid valve overlies portions of the septum. A sweep would help elucidate these structures. In the right panel, as the gain is increased, some artificial thickening of the left ventricular posterior wall is present due to excessive echoes. This echogram needs a bit more reject or damping.

Pertinent Measurements:

1. Right ventricular anterior wall = 0.23 cm.
2. Septum = 0.75 cm (> 95%).
3. Left ventricular posterior wall = 0.70 cm.
4. Right ventricular cavity = 2.1 cm (> 95%).
5. Left ventricular end diastolic dimension = 4.8 cm.
6. Vcf = 1.06 circumferences/sec (< 5%).

Clinical Comment:

Note that the wall measurements are the same as in the previous echocardiogram performed 1 week earlier.

The left ventricular cavity no longer is compressed by the effusion and its measurement now is normal. The right ventricular cavity still is slightly dilated. Now that the left ventricular compression has been relieved, myocarditis becomes a plausible explanation.

We still cannot explain the septal measurements exceeding the ninety-fifth percentile.

Pertinent literature references: see Chapter 3 and Chapter 4, Section 4.33.

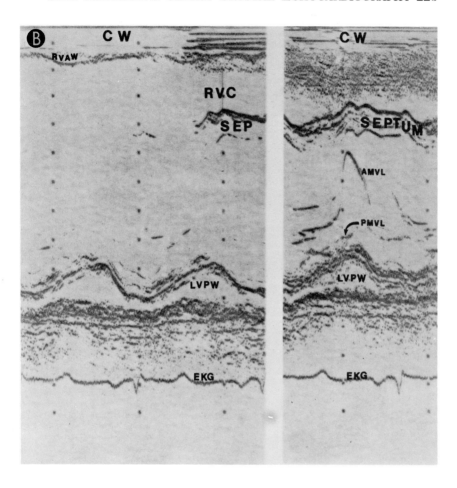

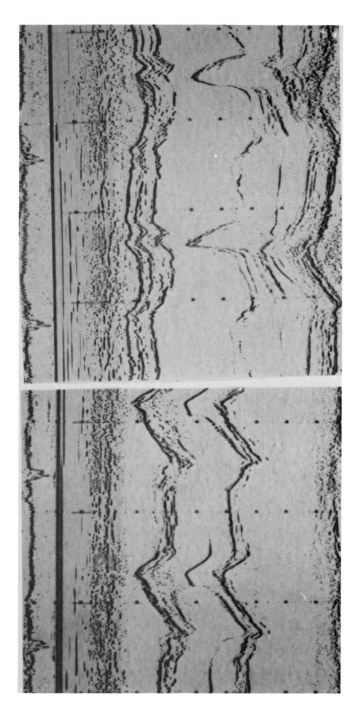

PROBLEM 11

This echocardiogram was performed on a 15-year-old boy with a body surface area of 1.5 m².

Reader's interpretation: _____

_____

_____

Measurements: _____

_____

_____

Diagnosis: _____

_____

_____

_____

This young man has congenital aortic stenosis and mild aortic insufficiency. Note that his aortic valve appears normal. During systole, fine fluttering of the opened leaflets frequently is found in normals and is believed to be induced by the echograph itself. Note that the aortic valve flutter occurs at exactly the same frequency as the flutter in the electrocardiogram. Careful measurement will confirm that the frequency is exactly 60 cycles/second. The diastolic closure line is eccentric.

The right-hand panel shows the main point of this echocardiogram. The left ventricular posterior wall and septum are concentrically hypertrophied at 0.9 cm in the plane of the posterior mitral valve leaflet. Note that although he has aortic insufficiency, no vibration of the anterior mitral valve leaflet was discernible.

Criticism of This Echocardiogram:

The right ventricular anterior wall is not seen clearly. Therefore, its measurement and right ventricular cavity measurement cannot be made in this view. On another area of this study, however, it was normal. Some fine echoes are present in each of these frames that could have been cleared with "fine tuning" of either the coarse gain or reject.

Pertinent Measurements:

1. Left atrium = 3.9 cm (> 95%).
2. Aortic dimension = 2.7 cm (> 95%).
3. Intercusp dimension = 1.7 cm.
4. Left ventricular end diastolic dimension = 5.3 cm (> 95%).
5. Left ventricular end systolic dimension (beat 1) = 3.0 cm.
6. Left ventricular posterior wall = 0.9 cm (> 95%).
7. Septum = 0.9 cm (> 95%).
8. Vcf = 1.36 circumferences/sec.

Clinical Comment:

A pressure load is imposed on the left ventricle with aortic stenosis. This accounts for the concentric hypertrophy. Aortic insufficiency presents a volume load that is accompanied by varying degrees of dilatation, depending on the amount of incompetence and the compliance and myocardial function of the ventricle. This patient has left ventricular dilatation exceeding the ninety-fifth percentile. Further, his Vcf is normal for an adult. Evidence of marginal ventricular decompensation is that the left atrium is dilated in the absence of a left-to-right shunt or mitral insufficiency. Finally, the aortic root exceeds the ninety-fifth percentile, which could be expected in aortic stenosis with insufficiency.

Pertinent literature references: see Chapter 4, Sections 4.7 and 4.8.

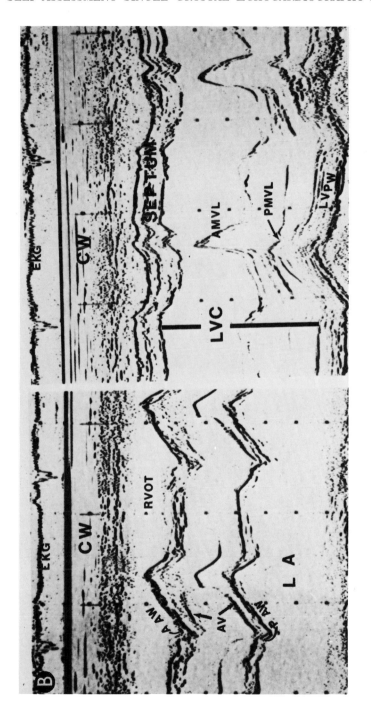

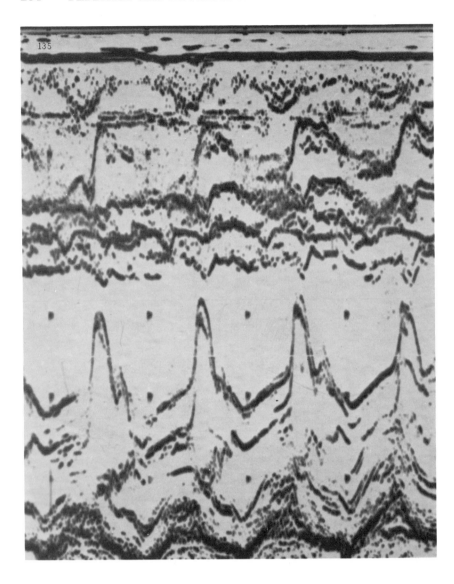

PROBLEM 12

The patient was a 4-year-old boy with a body surface area of 0.6 m².

Reader's interpretation: _____

_____

_____

Measurements: _____

_____

_____

Diagnosis: _____

_____

_____

_____

This boy's mother has idiopathic hypertrophic subaortic stenosis and he has mitral insufficiency and moderate elevation of pulmonary artery pressure.

This echocardiogram demonstrates asymmetric septal hypertrophy. The septal measurement is 0.8 cm with a left ventricular posterior wall measurement of 0.5 cm. The ratio of the septum to the left ventricular posterior wall in this instance is 1.78:1. The electrocardiogram runs through the middle of the septum, confusing septal measurement. Note that the tricuspid valve echo in beats 1 and 2 is adjacent to the septum. However, in beats 3 and 4 it clears the septum and the septum can be measured readily. Note also that the right ventricular anterior wall measures 2.5 mm; since the patient is not a neonate, this would make one think more in terms of familial asymmetric septal hypertrophy associated with the idiopathic hypertrophic subaortic stenosis syndrome.

Criticism of This Echocardiogram:

In the first few beats, the tricuspid valve echo could be confused with the septal echo. The electrocardiogram is in the middle of the septum. The right ventricular cavity is not clear.

Pertinent Measurements:

1. Right ventricular anterior wall = 0.25 cm.
2. Right ventricular cavity = 1.4 cm (> 95%).
3. Septum = 0.8 cm (> 95%).
4. Left ventricular posterior wall = 0.47 cm.
5. Septum/left ventricular posterior wall ratio = 1.78:1 (> 95%).
6. Left ventricular end diastolic dimension = 3.1 cm.

Clinical Comment:

Asymmetric septal hypertrophy is present, as discussed previously. The only other abnormal measurement in this echo is the right ventricular cavity exceeding the ninety-fifth percentile. Possibly this can be explained on the basis of his mild pulmonary hypertension. As the right ventricular anterior wall is not hypertrophied, the hypertension probably is not longstanding or severe.

Pertinent literature references: see Chapter 4, Section 4.10.

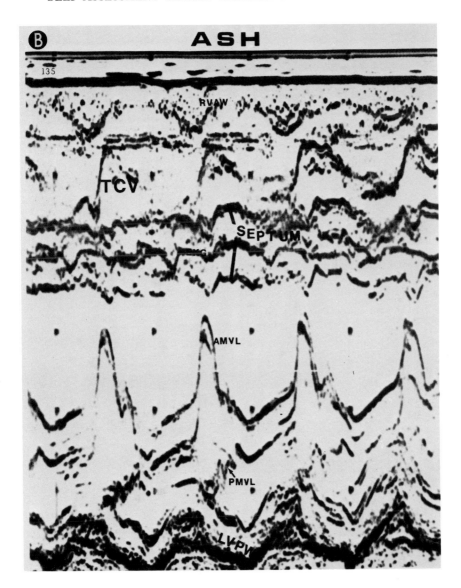

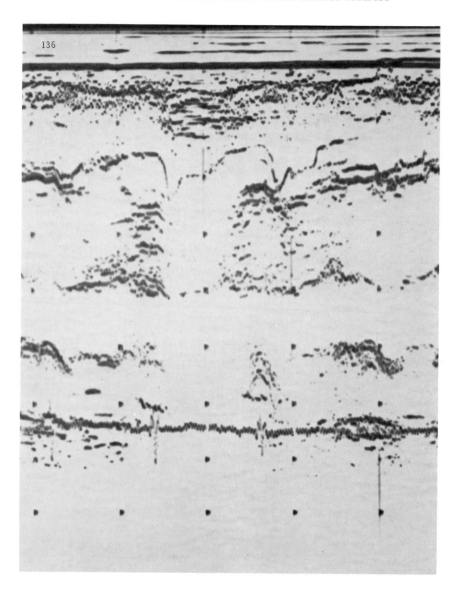

136

PROBLEM 13

This echocardiogram is from a 13-year-old girl with a body surface area of 0.9 m².

Reader's interpretation: _____

_____

_____

Measurements: _____

_____

_____

Diagnosis: _____

_____

_____

_____

This patient has a ventricular septal defect with pulmonary vascular obstructive disease. The echo is of the pulmonary valve (in this instance, the posterior pulmonary valve). Note that there is no presystolic posterior motion of the pulmonary valve following the P wave. Weyman et al.[233] and Gramiak et al.[89] suggested that this phenomenon was consistent with pulmonary vascular obstructive disease, and it indeed holds true in this patient. Soon after the valve opens, it drifts back toward closure rapidly rather than staying open fully throughout systole. This suggests high resistance in the lung circulation.

Criticism of This Echocardiogram:

The anterior pulmonary valve leaflet is not visualized. This is an angulation phenomenon (see Chapters 3 and 5).

Pertinent Measurements:

None can be made, as the anterior pulmonary valve leaflet is not visualized for intercusp distance, and the pulmonary root cannot be measured because it is not viewed in cross section.

Pertinent literature references: 89, 233.

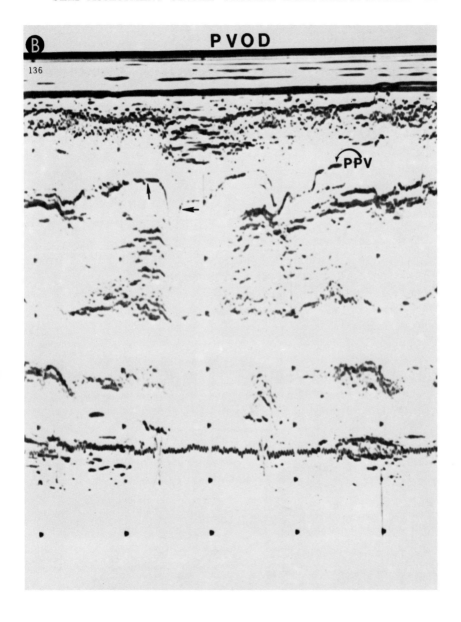

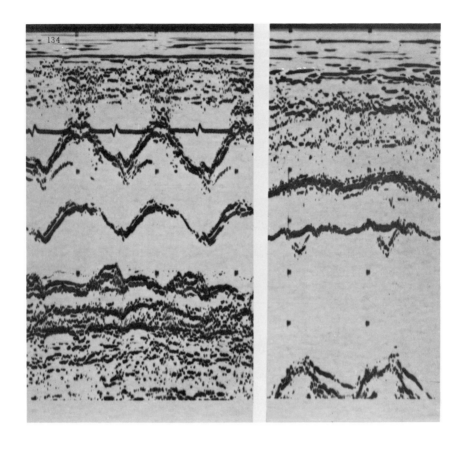

PROBLEM 14

This is an echocardiogram from a 6-month-old male with a body surface area of 0.3 m². Calibration markers are the same in each echo.

Reader's interpretation: _____

_____

_____

Measurements: _____

_____

_____

Diagnosis: _____

_____

_____

_____

Pectus excavatum causes a "pancaking" effect of the left atrium. The echocardiograms here are the Z axis (in the first panel) and the Y axis (in the second panel). The left atrial internal dimension is markedly increased in the Y dimension as compared with the Z dimension, reflecting this pancaking effect. This echocardiogram demonstrates the necessity for obtaining left atrial measurements in these two planes.

Criticism of This Echocardiogram:

The electrocardiogram is partially observed in the aorta. The aortic root is not clearly defined but can be measured.

Pertinent Measurements:

1. Anteroposterior:

   a) Z axis – aorta = 1.4 cm.

   b) Left atrial internal dimension = 1.4 cm.

2. Suprasternal notch:

   a) Y axis – ascending aorta = 1.4 cm. (Note that this is the same as the aortic measurement at the root.)

   b) Right pulmonary artery = 0.9 cm.

   c) Left atrial internal dimension = 3.0 cm.

Pertinent literature references: See Chapters 3 and 5.

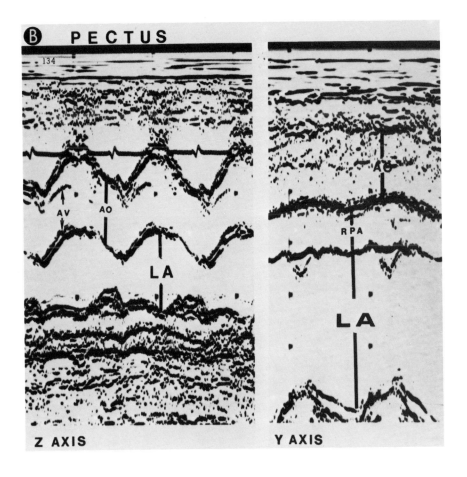

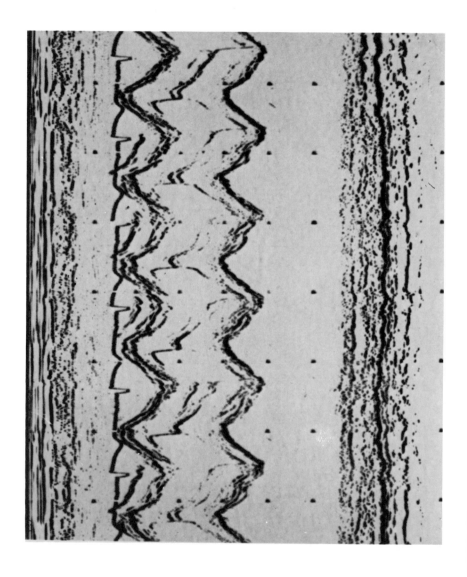

PROBLEM 15

The patient is a 6-year-old boy with a body surface area of 0.8 m².

Reader's interpretation: _____

_____

_____

Measurements: _____

_____

_____

Diagnosis: _____

_____

_____

_____

The patient has mild mitral insufficiency and a normal aortic valve demonstrated by catheterization and physical examination. The echocardiogram shows multiple diastolic closure lines and eccentricity of the diastolic closure in beats 3 and 6.

The left atrium is slightly dilated with respect to the aorta (left atrial dimension 2.8 cm, aortic dimension 2.5 cm). This is the secondary reflection of his mitral insufficiency.

Another Feature of This Echocardiogram:

The tricuspid echo is seen above the aorta in beats 1, 3, 4 and 5.

Pertinent Measurements:

1. Right ventricular outflow tract = 1.9 cm.

2. Intercusp distance = 1.5 cm.

Clinical Comment:

Caution! Do not overcall aortic stenosis on the basis of the echocardiogram.

Pertinent literature references: see Chapter 4, Sections 4.7 and 4.12.

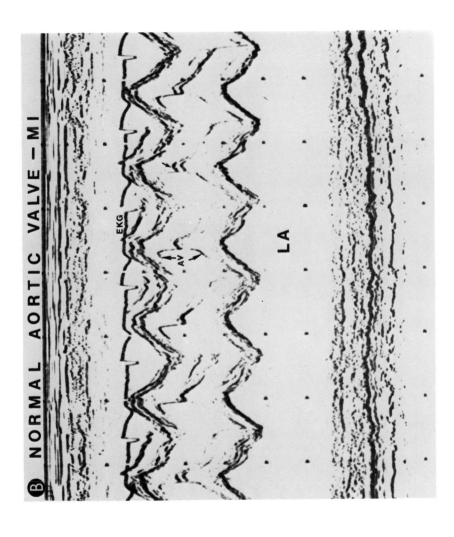

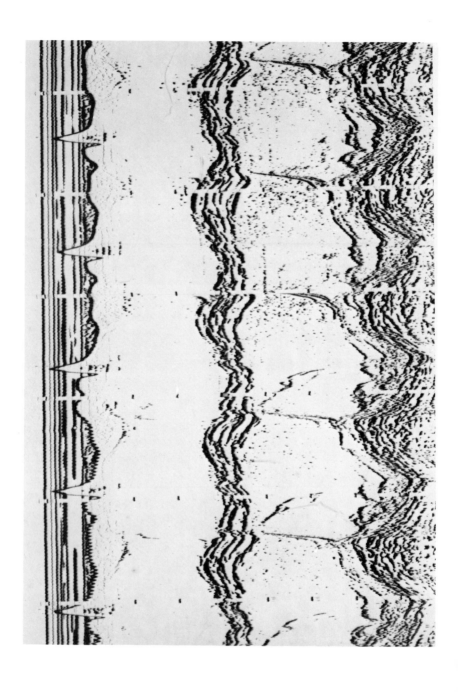

PROBLEM 16

The patient is a 7½-year-old female with a body surface area of 0.7 m². This and the following two problems were performed using a different echograph machine. Accordingly, the markers are displayed differently.

Reader's interpretation: _____

_____

_____

Measurements: _____

_____

_____

Diagnosis: _____

_____

_____

_____

A cardiac murmur was heard in this patient during a preoperative evaluation for a splenectomy because of chronically depressed platelet counts. The electrocardiogram suggested right ventricular hypertrophy. Increased pulmonary vascularity was present on the chest roentgenogram.

The two most interesting features on this echocardiogram are:

1. The significant increase in right ventricular dimension.

2. The abnormal motion of the septum in the region of the mitral valve.

Characteristics of this septal motion fulfill those described as Type II or Type B paradox with initial anterior motion in systole, followed by a terminal posterior motion. This would suggest right ventricular volume overload of modest degree and, indeed, the patient had an atrial septal defect with a Q_p/Q_s of 2.2:1. The evaluation of septal motion from a single echocardiographic view as this is treacherous, since the hinge point of the septum usually is found opposite the anterior mitral leaflet. Nevertheless, on the last three beats on the strip, the abnormality of septal motion persists as the transducer is angled farther into the ventricle.

The right ventricular anterior wall is visualized most clearly in the first three beats and a faint tricuspid valve echo may be seen within the right ventricle in that region. Mid- to late systolic prolapse of the mitral valve always should be searched for in patients with atrial septal defects; however, the systolic segments in the echocardiographic record are not seen well enough to make this observation.

Criticisms of This Echocardiogram:

1. In the evaluation of septal motion, a continuous sweep from the left ventricular body to the outflow tract should be obtained so that the motion of the septum may be viewed in various positions within the ventricular cavity.

2. The electrocardiogram trace as placed obscures the right ventricular anterior wall and makes it barely visible.

3. The mitral valve apparatus has not been well visualized, especially for the evaluation of systolic mitral valve motion.

Pertinent Measurements:

1. Left ventricular diastolic diameter = 3.4 cm.

2. Mitral valve excursion = 1.9 cm.

3. Right ventricular dimension = 2.6 cm (> 95%).

4. Septal thickness = 0.5 cm.

5. Posterior wall thickness = 0.55 cm.

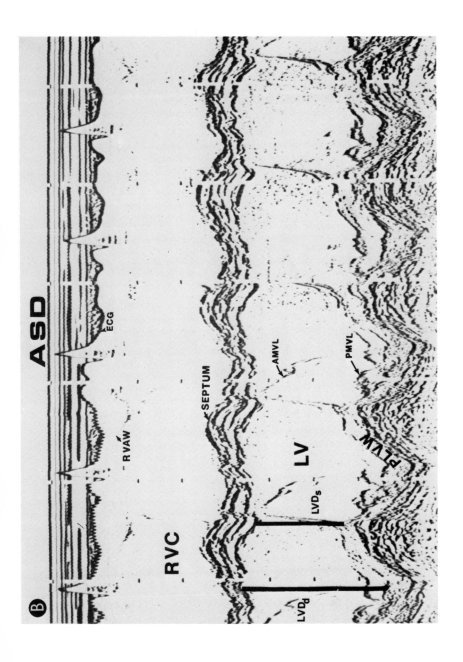

Clinical Comment:

Criteria often create problems. The septal motion pattern exhibited here appears closest to Type II or B with a septal motion pattern initially anterior in direction in early systole and then posterior. Nevertheless, considering the significant amplitude of the anterior motion, it appears very similar to Type A or true paradoxical septal motion. Septal motion definitely is abnormal as viewed and, on the basis of the limited sweep obtained, probably should not be classified further.

Pertinent literature references: see Chapter 4, Section 4.1.

NOTES

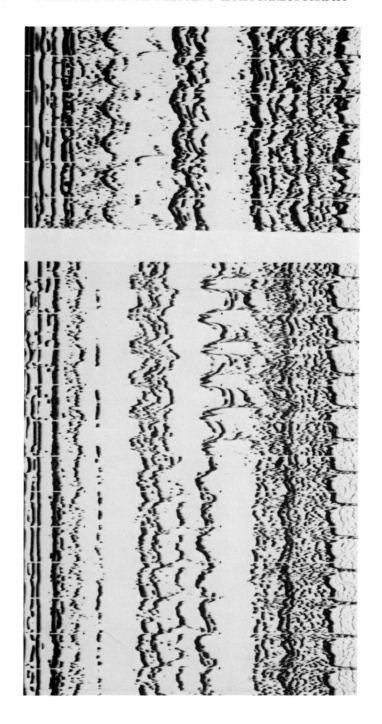

PROBLEM 17

The patient was a 6-pound term male infant with a body surface area of 0.2 m².

Reader's interpretation: _____

_____

_____

Measurements: _____

_____

_____

Diagnosis: _____

_____

_____

_____

Shortly after birth, this infant presented with cyanosis in the absence of signs of respiratory disease. X-ray examination revealed an increased cardiac size with nonspecifically increased lung markings. The infant was hypoxemic and acidotic, and congenital heart disease was suspected.

The echocardiogram demonstrates features of valve function. The mitral valve appears grossly normal, with normal motion of the anterior and posterior leaflets. The aortic valve, although not seen quite as well, opens for only a very short period in systole. The left ventricle, although of normal size, does not appear to contract vigorously and it would not seem that much blood is getting into or out of the left ventricle. At right, the pulmonary artery is visualized and is increased in dimension with normal valve structure. The pulmonary artery having been found to the left of the aorta rules out most forms of complete transposition.

The pattern visualized has been seen in some infants whom we have studied who have persistence of the fetal pathways of circulation. In such infants, most of the blood going out from the pulmonary artery achieves access to the descending aorta directly through a large patent ductus arteriosus and does not go to the lungs because of an increased residual pulmonary vascular resistance. Return of blood from the lungs to the left atrium and left ventricle is decreased, and most of the blood ejected from the left side of the heart is channeled directly into the vessels of the head. The echocardiogram rules out most serious forms of cyanotic congenital heart disease, and the mitral and aortic findings suggest decreased blood return to the left atrium and left ventricle as a physiologic sequel of the vascular resistance abnormality. Cardiac anatomy is normal in these infants.

Criticism of This Echocardiogram:

1. The left ventricular posterior wall has not been imaged adequately. The over-all quality of the echo in terms of the lack of gray scale and the poor interface definition might suggest the necessity for adjustment of the strip chart recording apparatus.

2. The tricuspid valve has not been demonstrated. A rightward angulation from the aortic position would have achieved this demonstration.

Pertinent Measurements:

1. Left ventricular diastolic dimension = 1.5 – 1.6 cm.
2. Left atrial dimension = 0.9 cm.
3. The aortic root dimension = 1.0 cm.
4. Right ventricular dimension = 1.1 cm.
5. Main pulmonary artery = 1.25 cm.

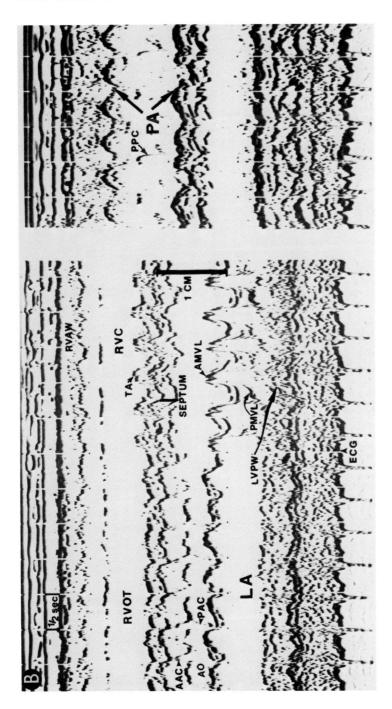

6. Septum = 0.25 cm.

7. Right ventricular anterior wall = 0.3 cm.

8. Left ventricular posterior wall is poorly defined and thickness could not be measured.

Clinical Comment:

The echoes present in the region of the septum contain tricuspid annulus tissue anterior to the right-sided septal interface. If this distance were included in measuring septal thickness, a false impression of asymmetric septal hypertrophy might result.

Pertinent literature references: See Chapter 3 and Chapter 4, Sections 4.2 and 4.22.

NOTES

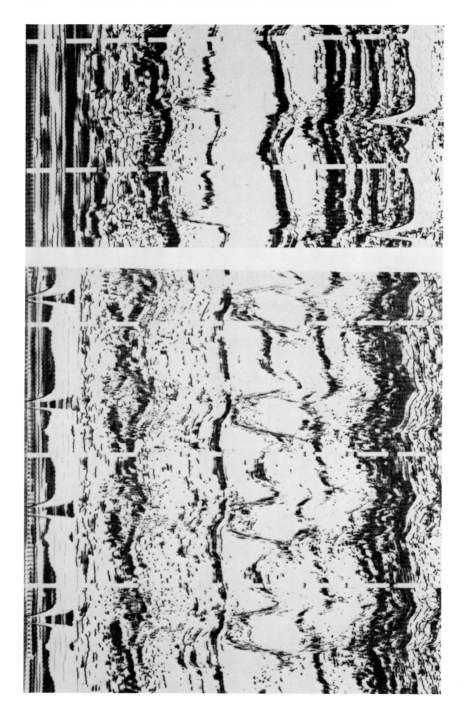

PROBLEM 18

The patient is a 9-year-old girl with a body surface area of 1 m².

Reader's interpretation: _____

_____

_____

Measurements: _____

_____

_____

Diagnosis: _____

_____

_____

_____

The patient had severe idiopathic hypertrophic subaortic stenosis (IHSS). A myotomy and myectomy (operative septal muscle resection) was performed. The echocardiogram was performed soon after operation.

The most striking feature of this echocardiogram is a marked increase in septal thickness. Posterior wall thickness is not clearly defined. The mitral valve continues to exhibit systolic anterior motion. No obvious pericardial effusion is present.

At right, the aortic root is imaged. It is significantly enlarged for a child in this weight range. Further, an anterior cusp in the aortic root exhibits a short period of opening early in systole, which is followed by premature closure. This finding has been described in both discrete subaortic stenosis and in idiopathic hypertrophic subaortic stenosis. The echocardiogram, therefore, suggests that the patient has residual outflow tract obstruction.

Another feature of general interest is that left atrial diameter as imaged is small. This is unusual for patients with significant left ventricular and septal hypertrophy.

Criticisms of This Echocardiogram:

1. At left, further damping of anterior structures would increase definition of the area of the right ventricle.

2. A more inferior section through the left ventricle probably would produce a better left ventricular endocardial echo.

3. At right, further angulation of the transducer toward the left probably would detect the posterior cusp of the aortic valve. Left atrial dimension might be measured more reliably if this were the case.

Pertinent Measurements:

1. At left, septal thickness = 2.1 cm (> 95%).

2. Posterior wall thickness cannot be measured.

3. Left ventricular diastolic dimension = approx 2.8 cm.

4. At right, aortic dimension = 3.1 cm (> 95%).

Clinical Comment:

A method has been described for estimating the outflow gradient in idiopathic hypertrophic subaortic stenosis based on an index of duration and distance of mitral valve to septal apposition (Section 4.10). This postoperative echocardiogram predicted a residual peak systolic gradient circa 20–35 mm Hg (85–120 mm Hg preoperatively).

Pertinent literature references: see Chapter 4, Section 4.10.

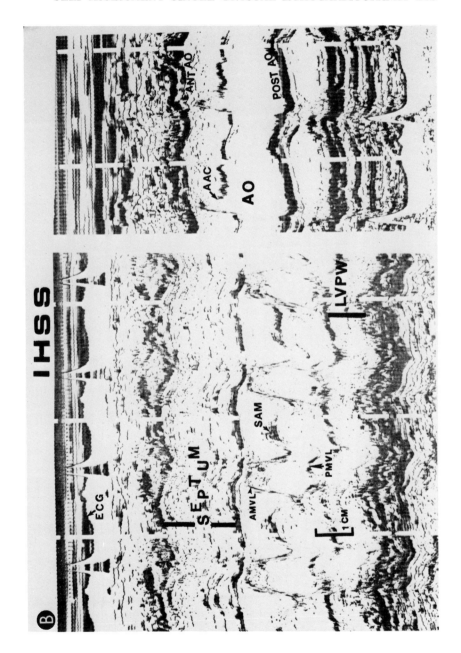

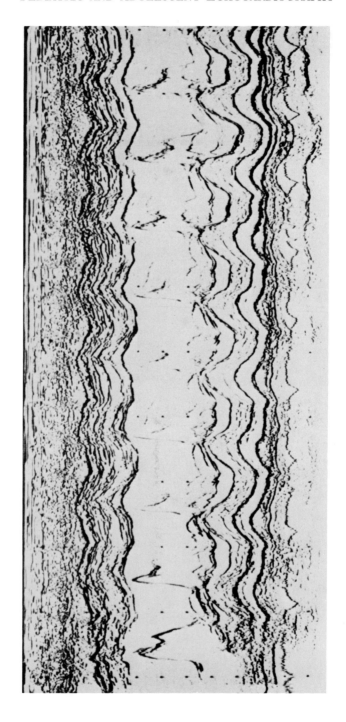

PROBLEM 19

The patient was a 4-year-old female with a body surface area of 0.5 m².

Reader's interpretation: _____

_____

_____

Measurements: _____

_____

_____

Diagnosis: _____

_____

_____

_____

The patient was a 4-year-old mongoloid female who had a cardiac catheterization at age 1 with a diagnosis of single ventricle. Subsequent catheterization with angiography showed a short stump of thickened septum superiorly and a septal rim near the apex. The entire membranous and most of the muscular septum was absent. QP:QS was 3.3:1. Aortic systolic pressure = pulmonary artery systolic pressure = ventricular systolic pressure = 80 mm Hg.

Because of the intracardiac anatomy and the high flow–high pressure pulmonary situation, a pulmonary artery banding procedure was performed. One week postoperatively, cardiac enlargement was noted on x-ray and the patient developed tachypnea and hepatomegaly.

The most striking feature of this echocardiogram is the posterior pericardial effusion. Note that the epicardium is separated from the dense pericardial echo. Usually these are represented by a single line. The effusion is demonstrated as a nearly echo-free space. However, this demonstration is a function of technique. The effusion can be missed with improper gain settings. Considerable experience, caution and careful technique are necessary to be certain of an effusion.

Note that the effusion disappears as the transducer is angled toward the aorta and left atrium (LA), beat 1. Proof that the beam enters the left atrium includes:

1. The posterior mitral valve leaflet (PMVL) disappears, but the anterior mitral valve leaflet (AMVL) remains.

2. The posterior wall in question is contracting prior to the QRS.

3. The left atrial wall is at a different depth than the posterior left ventricular wall.

4. The cavity sizes are different.

The septum is excessively thick in relation to the posterior left ventricular wall (PLVW). This could be considered asymmetric septal hypertrophy (ASH), but this patient had only a very small thick septum at catheterization. Asymmetric septal hypertrophy is not diagnosable when right ventricular hypertrophy coexists. This echo does not show the right ventricular wall clearly enough to measure and thus is unsuitable for determination of right ventricular hypertrophy. An approximation of right ventricular wall thickness is indicated on beat 1. If right ventricular hypertrophy were ruled out, asymmetric septal hypertrophy would be a consideration. Note the slight systolic anterior motion of the anterior mitral leaflet (beats 4 and 5). Systolic anterior motion, usually of greater magnitude, is a finding in idiopathic hypertrophic subaortic stenosis (IHSS). Could this systolic anterior motion be a function of unusual anatomy or secondary to pressure from the effusion in this patient?

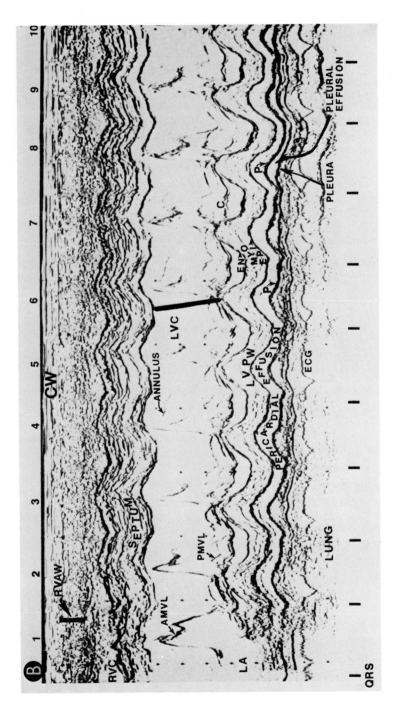

Other Features of This Echocardiogram:

1. In beats 7–10, a space between the pericardium and the pleura is demonstrated. This indicates a small pleural effusion.

2. Effusion is one of the few instances in which the epicardium is seen separate from the pericardium.

3. Chordae are visualized in the plane between the left ventricular posterior wall (LVPW) and posterior mitral valve leaflet.

4. The posterior mitral valve leaflet is seen best in beats 6–9 and moves away (posteriorly) from the anterior mitral valve leaflet during diastole and joins it to move anteriorly in systole.

5. In the 4th and 6th beats, elements that may be mitral valve ring are noted anterior to the anterior mitral valve leaflet. These must not be confused with systolic anterior motion or idiopathic hypertrophic subaortic stenosis.

6. This study is a particularly good example of left ventricular contraction. Note that the septum moves posteriorly before the left ventricular wall contracts. This is shown with a slightly diagonal line in beat 6.

Criticisms of This Echocardiogram:

1. The electrocardiogram would be visualized better if it were placed farther below the echo.

2. The anterior right ventricular wall is not demonstrated clearly. A decrease in anterior gain might have improved the tracing quality.

3. Ideally, one would attempt to show the aorta and its valve on this strip.

Pertinent Measurements:

1. Left ventricular posterior wall thickness = 0.85 cm (> 95%).
2. Left ventricular cavity, end diastole = 4.2 cm (> 95%).
3. Left ventricular cavity, systole = 2.75 cm (> 95%).
4. Septum = 2.0 cm (> 95%).
5. Right ventricular wall = approximately 1.1 cm (> 95%).
6. Left atrium cannot be measured in this view.

Clinical Comment:

This patient has an unusual rim of septum. Criteria for asymmetric septal hypertrophy should not be applied to this situation. Criteria for right ventricular hypertrophy probably are present also. In this instance, it may be improper to compare ventricular dimensions with normals, for the patient had a nearly single ventricle. Additionally, we frequently see thickened ventricular septum in patients with endocardial cushion defects.

Pertinent literature references: see Chapter 4, Sections 4.5 and 4.33.

7 / Cross-Sectional Echocardiography in the Evaluation of Congenital Heart Disease

CROSS-SECTIONAL ECHOCARDIOGRAPHY is an advance in diagnostic ultrasound that has great potential for noninvasive evaluation of intracardiac and extracardiac structural relationships. Several types are in use. These include (1) stop-action B scan,[129] (2) single crystal scanners[93] and (3) multicrystal arrays.[14-16, 135, 193, 196, 197]

If one were searching a dark room for a companion, would one be more likely to find him with one or with twenty flashlights? Cross-sectional echocardiography is an approach to noninvasive diagnosis that seeks to answer questions of spatial orientation by providing multiple simultaneous views of cardiac anatomy.

STOP-ACTION CARDIAC ULTRASONOGRAPHY

Stop-action cardiac ultrasonography is a technique similar to the B scan echo performed for abdominal examinations. A two-dimensional stop-action image of a section through the heart is formed by composite multiple sequential B scan recordings produced by slowly moving the ultrasound transducer of a contact scanner along a predetermined path that sections the heart. A storage oscilloscope is triggered by the electrocardiogram so that echoes are recorded from each point in the section at an identical time in the cardiac cycle.[129]

REAL-TIME CROSS-SECTIONAL METHODS

A real-time motion adaptation of this technique is obtained by a single crystal that is mechanically swept through a sector arc. Its angular position is transmitted to the oscilloscope so that echoes returning during any portion of the angular sweep are placed in their appropriate geographic locations. A 25° to 45° sector may be scanned at a sweep repetition rate of 30–50 cycles/sec. These sweep speeds are sufficiently rapid to cause the displayed image to appear to move in real time.[93] This technique is quite new and may assume great importance.

The majority of our experience has been with a multicrystal echo-

271

cardiographic system designed by Bom.[14-16, 135, 193, 196, 197] Twenty parallel single-element brightness-modulated lines are displayed sequentially from the twenty crystals in the 8-cm-long transducer. Each element transmits a short acoustic pulse in sequence into the tissues and receives the returning energy before activation of the next element. Echoes are displayed on the oscilloscope so that depth of the structure is indicated on the horizontal axis and crystal element lines are on the vertical to correspond to the geographic position of the respective element in the transducer array (Fig. 7-1). The system produces cross-sectional images at a frame rate of 160/sec. If lines are duplicated by an interlacing technique, 40 lines may be displayed at an effective frame rate of 80/sec and a real-time cross-sectional echocardiographic study is provided. Simultaneous patient identification information and an ECG trace are also displayed.

Despite differences in approach to cross-sectional echocardiography, the same congenital cardiac lesion will appear similarly by each technique. The following summary will relate our approach to elucidation of intracardiac and extracardiac spatial relationships with Bom's technique. Pertinent examples of cardiac abnormalities will be included. It must be appreciated that illustrations that accompany this chapter are single frames derived from real-time motion studies that are best visualized on an oscilloscope. Furthermore, they have been subjected to photographic enlargement from a small-format motion picture film. A few were derived from ECG gated Polaroid

Fig. 7-1.—Schematic drawing of the layout of the multi-element transducer and the oscilloscopic display obtained from a cylindrical target. (Courtesy of Dr. N. Bom and Biomedical Engineering 6:500, 1971.)

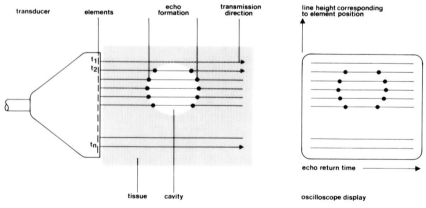

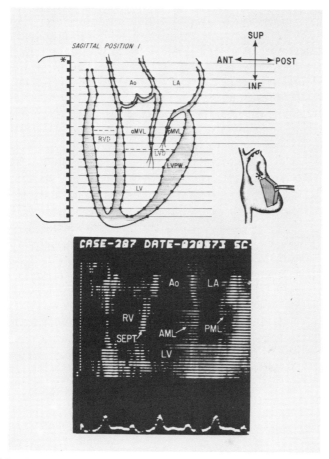

Fig. 7-2.—Position 1: Normal sagittal cross section. The top of the transducer (indicated by the asterisk) is superior. The lower panel is a Polaroid photograph. Mitral aortic and septal continuity are shown. *Ao* = aorta; *LA* = left atrium; *AML, aMVL* = anterior mitral valve leaflet; *PML, pMVL* = posterior mitral valve leaflet; *LV* = left ventricle; *RV* = right ventricle; *LVPW* = left ventricular posterior wall; *RVD* and *LVD* represent areas where ventricular dimensions would be measured. (By permission of the American Heart Association, Inc. Sahn, D. J., Terry, R., O'Rourke, R., and Friedman, W. F.: Multiple crystal cross-sectional echocardiography in the diagnosis of cyanotic congenital heart disease, Circulation 50:230, 1974.)

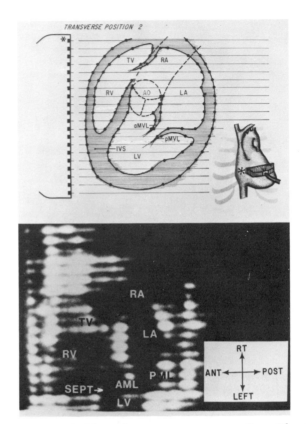

Fig. 7-3.—Position 2: Normal transverse cross section. The top of the transducer (indicated by the asterisk) is toward the right. The lower section is a still frame selected from an 8-mm motion picture. In this cross section, right and left ventricular anatomy is seen. Tilting the transducer superiorly demonstrates the aortic root (vertical dashed lines). *AO* = aorta; *LA* = left atrium; *AML, aMVL* = anterior mitral valve leaflets; *PML, pMVL* = posterior mitral valve leaflets; *LV* = left ventricle; *IVS, SEPT* = interventricular septum; *RV* = right ventricle; *TV* = tricuspid valve; *RA* = right atrium. (By permission of the American Heart Association, Inc. Sahn, D. J., Terry, R., O'Rourke, R., and Friedman, W. F.: Multiple crystal cross-sectional echocardiography in the diagnosis of cyanotic congenital heart disease, Circulation 50:230, 1974.)

prints. Anatomic details are substantially clearer on the oscilloscope, and identification is facilitated by viewing the moving images.

Cross-sectional cardiac anatomy is evaluated in a systematic manner in our laboratory. We use two sagittal and two transverse views as follows.[196, 197]

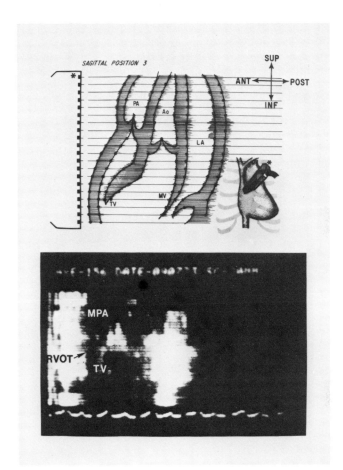

Fig. 7-4.—Position 3: Sagittal section along the line of the right ventricular outflow tract. The lower panel is a still frame selected from an 8-mm motion picture. The top of the transducer (indicated by the asterisk) is superior and toward the left shoulder. The normal posterior sweep of the main pulmonary artery is shown. The interventricular septum is not visualized in this position. *LA* = left atrium; *Ao* = aorta; *PA, MPA* = main pulmonary artery; *TV* = tricuspid valve; *MV* = mitral valve; *RVOT* = right ventricular outflow tract. (By permission of the American Heart Association, Inc. Sahn, D. J., Terry, R., O'Rourke, R., and Friedman, W. F.: Multiple crystal cross-sectional echocardiography in the diagnosis of cyanotic congenital heart disease, Circulation 50:230, 1974.)

Position 1 — Sagittal: The transducer is placed vertically along the left sternal border in the long axis of the heart (Fig. 7-2).

Position 2 — Transverse: The transducer is placed horizontally in the fourth intercostal space just to the left of the sternum (Fig. 7-3).

Position 3 — Modified Sagittal: The transducer is placed obliquely with the bottom element in the third intercostal space at the left sternal border and the top element below the left clavicle (Fig. 7-4).

Fig. 7-5. — Position 4: Transverse section showing normal great vessel orientation in the second intercostal space. The top of the transducer (indicated by the asterisk) is toward the right. The lower panel is a still frame selected from an 8-mm motion picture. The pulmonary artery is to the left of and anterior to the aorta. *Ao* = aorta; *PA, Pul* = pulmonary artery; *RVOT* = right ventricular outflow tract; *IVS* = interventricular septum; *LA* = left atrium. (By permission of the American Heart Association, Inc. Sahn, D. J., Terry, R., O'Rourke, R., and Friedman, W. F.: Multiple crystal cross-sectional echocardiography in the diagnosis of cyanotic congenital heart disease, Circulation 50:230, 1974.)

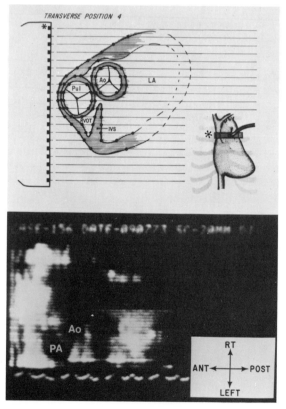

Position 4—Transverse: The transducer is placed horizontally in the second intercostal space (Fig. 7-5).

The position of cardiac structures when viewed in this format will be reviewed.

NORMAL ANATOMY

POSITION 1—SAGITTAL VIEW OF THE HEART IN THE LONG AXIS (Fig. 7-2).—The right ventricle and right ventricular outflow tract occupy the anterior superior portion of the section. The septum is continuous with the anterior wall of the aorta. The anterior and posterior walls of the aorta are parallel and the anterior mitral leaflet is a direct inferior extension of the posterior aortic wall. The anchoring of the anterior mitral valve leaflet by its chordae tendineae to the anterior papillary muscle may be visualized in some patients. The left atrium is posterior to the aorta. The position of the mitral annulus, which gives rise to the posterior mitral leaflet, is visualized at the atrioventricular junction. Below this is the left ventricular wall.

POSITION 2—TRANSVERSE.—In this position (Fig. 7-3), a transverse section through the body of the ventricles is obtained at the fourth intercostal space. In this and in Position 4, the top of the transducer is to the right. The right-sided structures will appear at the top of the cross-sectional image. The tricuspid valve and annulus lie at the most rightward anterior portion of the cross section. The right atrium is visualized posteriorly. The interatrial septum is not visualized, as it lies almost parallel to the ultrasound incident beams. Likewise, the ventricular septum is only partially visualized in this view. An oblique section of the right ventricular cavity, bounded by the anterior portion of the ventricular septum, lies leftward and anterior to the tricuspid valve. The mitral annulus and anterior mitral leaflet are posterior to the septum and are separated from it by the width of the left ventricular outflow tract. The left posterior portion of the cardiac section is composed of the posterior mitral leaflet and the posterior left ventricular wall. Left and right ventricular dimensions may be measured in this view (Fig. 7-3) and closely correspond to similar measurements obtained in Sagittal Position 1 (Fig. 7-2). Tilting the transducer superiorly from the position shown scans the left ventricular outflow tract and demonstrates mitral-aortic and septal-aortic continuity (Fig. 7-3).

POSITION 3—SAGITTAL.—In this position, the transducer is aligned along the right ventricular outflow tract (Fig. 7-4). The septal leaflet of the tricuspid valve is visualized best below the infundibulum.

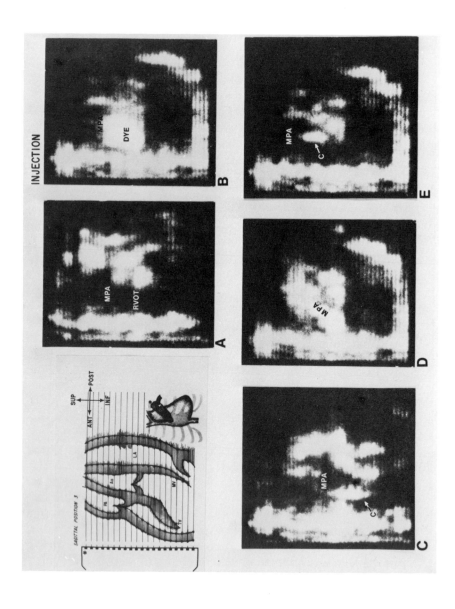

Fig. 7-6.—Visualization of passage of dye injected into the right ventricular outflow tract. Position 3, Sagittal. The line drawing (*top left*) shows the orientation of structures in this plane. Subsequent panels from an 8-mm motion picture follow from **A** through **E** the echoes produced by an injection of indocyanine green dye into the right ventricular outflow tract (*RVOT*). In panel **D** echoes are seen traversing the main pulmonary artery (*MPA*). The normal posterior sweep of the *MPA* is well demonstrated. The catheter (*C*) produces artifacts seen in lower panels **C** and **E**. *Ao* = aorta; *LA* = left atrium; *TV* = tricuspid valve; *MV* = mitral valve.

The right ventricular outflow tract sweeps posteriorly and pulmonary cusp tissue marks the position of this valve. The aorta passes obliquely from left to right and is partially seen in cross section.

POSITION 4—TRANSVERSE.—In this position, normal great vessel orientation may be viewed with the transducer in the second intercostal space (Fig. 7-5). The top of the transducer is to the right. The pulmonary artery is to the left of and anterior to the aorta. Thus, the pulmonary artery is seen at the bottom of the multiscan cross section. Cusp tissue within this anterior vessel may be found by tilting the transducer slightly superiorly, whereas cusp tissue within the posterior vessel may be found by tilting the transducer slightly inferiorly.

These cardiac cross sections are not routinely used angiographically and rarely are found in anatomy textbooks. Moreover, no precedent exists for the types of echoes displayed in these studies. Therefore it was necessary to validate echo identification of intracardiac and extracardiac structures in these four cross-sectional planes. This aim was achieved by viewing catheter echoes and passage of indocyanine green dye in known chambers with the multiscan technique during hemodynamic studies.[198] As an illustration of this validation technique, two views of the pulmonary artery are included in Figure 7-6. In this illustration, the identification of the main pulmonary artery in Sagittal Position 3 was verified by sighting a catheter. Further, an injection of indocyanine green dye into the right ventricular outflow tract produced selective echo opacification and showed the posterior sweep of the main pulmonary artery.

The transducer may be placed superiorly along the line of the left ventricular outflow tract so that it follows the course of the ascending aorta. This allows evaluation of the position and diameter of the ascending aorta. Even though the ascending aorta passes to the right behind the sternum, adequate visualization still may be obtained in young children. Supravalvular aortic constriction or poststenotic dilatation of the ascending aorta can be seen in this view.

The information assembled in these four views allows the construction of a three-dimensional model of cardiac anatomy. Quantitative measurement may be obtained from appropriate recordings.

Single crystal recordings in M-mode may be obtained from any of the crystals in the twenty-crystal array for accurate hard copy measurements.[193] Table 7-1 is a multicrystal echocardiographic check list detailing observations that should be made routinely. Each observation usually can be recorded during a single examination. Most studies have been performed with a 4.5-MHz transducer in children

TABLE 7-1. — MULTICHANNEL ECHOCARDIOGRAM WORKSHEET

Name_____ No._____ Date_____ MS No._____

Age_____ Dx_____

SEPTUM   Measure: V_____   [   ]   H_____   [   ]
      Motion: Normal_____ Paradoxical_____
      Septal-Aortic Continuity: Present_____ Absent_____ Not Seen_____

LEFT VENTRICLE   Measure: V_____   [   ]   H_____   [   ]
               Motion:_____
               Effusion: None_____ Ant._____ Post._____

LV OUTFLOW   Measure: V_____   [   ]

AORTA   Measure: At Cusps   V_____   [   ]   H_____   [   ]
      Above Valve   V_____   [   ]
      Cusps   Seen_____ D_____ S_____   Not Seen_____

LEFT ATRIUM   Measure: V_____   [   ]

MITRAL VALVE   Visualized: Ant. Leaflet_____ Post. Leaflet_____
           Excursion:_____   [   ]
           Post. Leaflet Motion: Normal_____ Abnormal_____
           Mitral-Aortic Continuity: Seen_____ Not Seen_____
           Dx: MS_____ MR_____ Prolapse_____ SAM_____ Normal_____

RIGHT VENTRICLE   Measure: V_____   [   ]   H_____   [   ]

PULMONARY ARTERY   Measure: V_____   [   ]   H_____   [   ]
               Cusps: Seen_____ S_____ D_____   Not Seen_____

TRICUSPID VALVE   Visualized_____ V_____ H_____
            Excursion_____   [   ]

RIGHT ATRIUM   Measure: V_____   [   ]   H_____   [   ]

GREAT VESSEL ORIENTATION   Normal_____ Abnormal_____

V = Vertical (Sagittal)
H = Horizontal (Transverse)

over 15 pounds. For patients under this weight, a commercially available 7-MHz (5 cm) transducer probably is more suitable. Multi-crystal echocardiographic criteria evolved for the abnormalities detailed in Table 7-2 will be discussed.

TABLE 7–2. – Multiscan Diagnoses

I. Mitral Valve
   A. Mitral stenosis
   B. Mitral regurgitation
   C. Endocardial cushion defect
II. Aortic Valve
   A. Valvular aortic stenosis, aortic insufficiency
   B. Supravalvular aortic stenosis
   C. Discrete subvalvular aortic stenosis
   D. IHSS
   E. Hypoplastic left heart
III. Tricuspid Valve
   A. Tricuspid atresia
   B. Ebstein's anomaly
IV. Pulmonic Valve
   A. Valvular pulmonic stenosis
V. Right Ventricular Volume Overload
VI. Great Vessel Relationships
   A. Tetralogy of Fallot
   B. Truncus arteriosus
   C. D-Transposition of the great vessels
   D. L-Transposition ("corrected" transposition)
   E. Double outlet right ventricle
VII. Single Ventricle

ABNORMALITIES STUDIED BY THE MULTICRYSTAL TECHNIQUE

Mitral Valve Disorders

MITRAL STENOSIS. – Cross-sectional findings in congenital mitral stenosis are similar to those described for older individuals by single crystal echo.[45] The child's posterior leaflet is somewhat more easily identified in cross-sectional examination. Major criteria include: a thickened mitral leaflet and/or multiple echoes and simultaneous diastolic anterior motion of the anterior and posterior mitral leaflets. In real time, this usually is seen as a sudden jerking motion that is easily distinguished from normal.

MITRAL INSUFFICIENCY. – The characteristics of mitral insufficiency include an increased excursion of the mitral leaflet with left atrial and/or left ventricular dilatation. In either rheumatic carditis or SBE, the mitral leaflet may be thickened relative to its annulus and chordal suspension. In the presence of mitral valve prolapse of the click-murmur type,[126, 179, 180] excessive mobility of the mitral leaflet may be accompanied by arching of the leaflet on its suspension as shown in Figure 7-7 or obvious prolapse into the left atrial cavity.

ENDOCARDIAL CUSHION DEFECT. – Endocardial cushion defect presents a spectrum of congenital heart disease starting with the os-

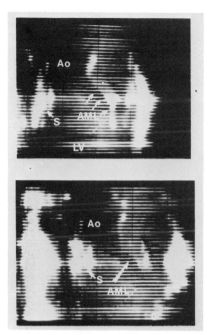

Fig. 7-7.—Two Polaroid still frames in a single patient illustrate the systolic arching of the anterior mitral valve leaflet *(AML)* (sagittal view) seen in patients with mitral valve prolapse. A concave arch is formed by the leaflet tissue. The posterior mitral valve leaflet is apposed to the posterior left ventricular wall, and though poorly defined, it is visible in the upper panel. *Ao* = aorta; *S* = septum; *LV* = left ventricle.

tium primum atrial septal defect with or without ventricular septal defect to complete atrioventricular canal. Most variants have an abnormal anchoring of the anterior inferior portion of the anterior mitral leaflet caused by an absence of the atrioventricular portion of the cardiac septum. As such, there is a shift in the position of the orifice of the mitral valve toward the right side of the left ventricle and a rotation of the orifice into the sagittal plane.[8, 176, 235] The leaflets may have anomalous chordal attachments and clefting. The abnormality of the mitral valve therefore is the most useful indicator of this abnormality. Major criteria for diagnosis of endocardial cushion defect include: (1) decreased mitral excursion, which is almost entirely anterior in direction toward the septum, with diastolic anterior mitral leaflet-septal apposition, (2) the presence of multiple echoes within the mitral leaflet area (Fig. 7-8, A) and (3) passage of the leaflet tissue across the ventricular septum into the right ventricular cavity in pa-

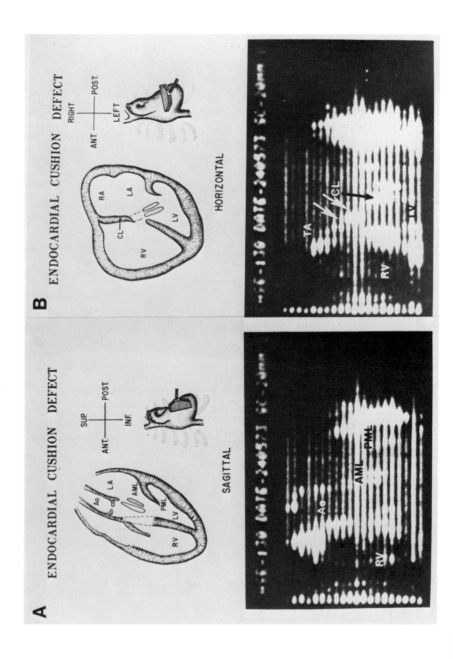

Fig. 7-8.–A, Position 1: Sagittal section in complete atrioventricular canal. Diagram and still frame show multiple echoes in the mitral valve area. A prominent posterior mitral valve leaflet and enlarged right ventricular cavity are seen. RV = right ventricle; LV = left ventricle; LA = left atrium; AML = anterior mitral valve leaflet; PML = posterior mitral valve leaflet. **B,** Position 2: Transverse (horizontal) section in complete atrioventricular canal. Diagram and still frame show multiple echoes (arrows) in the mitral valve area, right ventricular enlargement and the relationship of the common leaflet to the tricuspid valve annulus in a patient with complete atrioventricular canal. RV = right ventricle; LV = left ventricle; RA = right atrium; LA = left atrium; CL = common leaflet; TA = tricuspid annulus. (By permission of the American Heart Association, Inc. Sahn, D. J., Terry, R., O'Rourke, R., Leopold, G., and Friedman, W. F.: Multiple crystal echocardiographic evaluation of endocardial cushion defect, Circulation 50:25, 1974.)

tients with complete AV canal (Fig. 7-9). This sign is the most assuring diagnostically. Further, on transverse section, as visualized in Figure 7-8, *B*, the anterior mitral leaflet may appear to be an extension of a large common leaflet that is related to both the tricuspid annulus and the mitral annulus. Patients with this lesion who have a significant left-to-right atrial or ventricular shunt may have significant volume overload of the right ventricle. They may exhibit true paradoxical septal motion. Nonspecific findings include increased right ventricular dimension and increased pulmonary artery size.

Left Ventricular Outflow Tract Abnormalities

Multiscan Position 1 permits continued visualization of the left ventricular outflow tract above the aortic valve and allows complete evaluation of the anatomy of the left ventricular outflow tract.

VALVULAR AORTIC STENOSIS. — As discussed in Chapter 4, the single crystal echocardiographic description of the congenitally deformed aortic valve has been unreliable. It is difficult to define asymmetric positioning of the orifice and restricted opening of the valve cusps.[165] As illustrated in Figure 7-10, *A*, echo beams passing through the base of a domed aortic valve may fail to detect the stenotic orifice while the leaflets at their insertion appear to move laterally to a position of complete opening. We examined 15 patients with congenital aortic stenosis. Eighty per cent had detectable poststenotic dilatation of the ascending aorta as viewed in sagittal section, even in the presence of mild obstruction. In 55% of the patients examined, the time-motion study revealed that the leaflets had an excessive superior-inferior excursion or poor lateral mobility. Both are the cross-sectional echocardiographic equivalents of leaflet doming. The appearance of the left ventricular outflow tract in one of these patients is seen in Figure 7-10, *B*.

SUPRAVALVULAR AORTIC STENOSIS. — In supravalvular aortic stenosis, an hourglass configuration of the ascending aorta above the sinuses of Valsalva was seen in 9 of 10 patients. In the other patient, the narrowing was so close to the aortic valve that it was not detectable as a supravalvular deformity. It must be cautioned that the echocardiographic visualization of this deformity usually underestimates the angiographic survey, since there usually is considerable endothelial thickening in this disease (Fig. 7-11).

DISCRETE SUBVALVULAR AORTIC STENOSIS. — The single crystal echocardiographic findings in discrete subvalvular aortic stenosis were the subject of a recent report.[185] A discrete thickened area of the

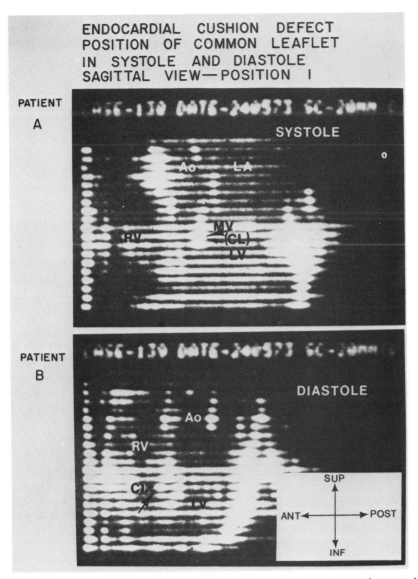

ENDOCARDIAL CUSHION DEFECT
POSITION OF COMMON LEAFLET
IN SYSTOLE AND DIASTOLE
SAGITTAL VIEW—POSITION I

Fig. 7-9.—Position 1: Sagittal section; complete atrioventricular canal. Still-frame examples from 2 patients of multiple echoes in the mitral valve area with common leaflet *(CL)* located within the left ventricle during systole *(top panel—arrow)* and in the right ventricle during diastole *(bottom panel— arrow)*. The right ventricle is enlarged in both patients. *RV* = right ventricle; *Ao* = aorta; *LV* = left ventricle; *LA* = left atrium; *MV* = mitral valve. (By permission of the American Heart Association, Inc. Sahn, D. J., Terry, R., O'Rourke, R., Leopold, G., and Friedman, W. F.: Multiple crystal echocardiographic evaluation of endocardial cushion defect, Circulation 50:25, 1974.)

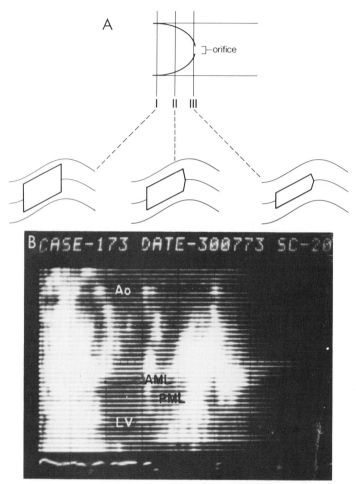

Fig. 7-10.—**A,** In the presence of a domed aortic valve, the systolic echographic appearance of the aortic valve leaflet is dependent on the portion of the dome subtended by the beam as shown in planes 1, 2 and 3 with corresponding aortic valve illustrations. **B,** A sagittal view of the left ventricular outflow tract is visualized in a patient with mild aortic stenosis. In this systolic frame, the aortic valve cusp tissue, as visualized, has moved superiorly within the aortic root but remains located in the central lumen (a sign of doming). The anterior wall of the ascending aorta is bowed forward (poststenotic dilatation). *Ao* = aorta; *LV* = left ventricle; *AML* = anterior mitral leaflet; *PM* = posterior mitral leaflet.

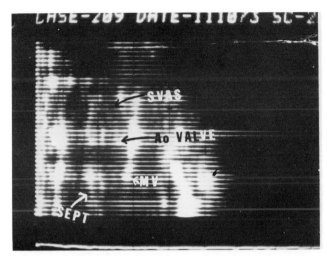

Fig. 7-11.—The echocardiographic findings in supravalvular aortic stenosis as viewed in the sagittal plane are illustrated with a polaroid still. In the photograph, the area designated *SVAS* denotes a narrowing of the aorta above the level of the aortic valve. There is poststenotic dilatation distal (superior) to this region. *SEPT* = septum; *Ao VALVE* = aortic valve; *MV* = anterior mitral valve.

septum beneath the aortic valve was visualized in Sagittal Position 1 (Fig. 7-12) in all 6 of our patients. The septal bulge seems to narrow the left ventricular outflow tract, but the systolic anterior motion of IHSS is not seen. Three of our 6 patients with subaortic stenosis had considerable poststenotic dilatation of the ascending aorta and 2 had abnormally thickened aortic valve leaflets. A mitral valve abnormality sometimes is present in patients with this lesion. In the illustration shown, both mitral leaflets were anchored to an enlarged papillary muscle in a pattern characteristic of mitral stenosis, secondary to a parachute deformity of the mitral valve.

IDIOPATHIC HYPERTROPHIC SUBAORTIC STENOSIS.—The findings visualized in idiopathic hypertrophic subaortic stenosis are similar to those described in single crystal echo papers.[183, 205] There is uniformly increased asymmetric septal thickening, more striking than in concentric ventricular hypertrophy. The septal bulge impinges on the left ventricular outflow tract and the systolic anterior motion of the mitral valve may be visualized in the sagittal or horizontal cross section. The detail of left ventricular outflow tract obstruction ob-

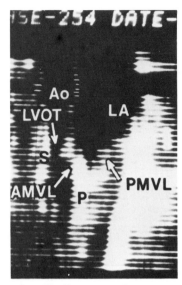

Fig. 7-12.—A Polaroid still illustrates the anterior mitral valve leaflet *(AMVL)* and the posterior mitral valve leaflet *(PMVL)*, which, in this patient, are anchored to a single papillary muscle *(P)*, constituting the parachute mitral valve deformity. Further, there is narrowing of the left ventricular outflow tract by a concentric ring visualized on the septum and mitral annulus in the area designated *LVOT*. Thickening is seen mainly on the mitral side. *Ao* = aortic root; *S* = septum; *LA* = left atrium.

tained with the multiscan technique in Sagittal Position 1 is quite similar to the lateral angiographic view (Fig. 7-13).

HYPOPLASTIC LEFT HEART SYNDROME.—As with single crystal studies in newborn infants with variations of the hypoplastic left heart syndrome, cross-sectional echocardiography may display hypoplasia or absence of a detectable mitral valve echo and/or hypoplasia of the ascending aorta with a diminutive left ventricular cavity.[153] The ease of orientation and rapid identification of a single AV valve in these infants makes the diagnosis.

Tricuspid Valve

EBSTEIN'S ANOMALY.—A variety of abnormal leaflet findings have been visualized by single crystal echocardiography in Ebstein's anomaly of the tricuspid valve.[141] The majority of these findings represent abnormalities of valve function rather than the basic defect of valve position and structure. In our 5 patients, multiple tricuspid

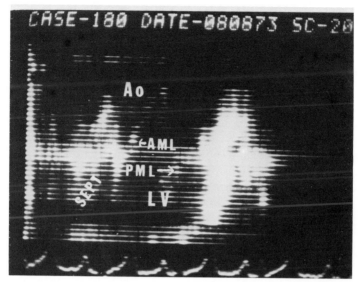

Fig. 7-13.—A sagittal view shows a septal bulge in a patient with idiopathic hypertrophic subaortic stenosis (IHSS). The panel is a Polaroid still. *Ao* = aorta; *PML* = posterior mitral valve leaflet; *LV* = left ventricle.

valve leaflet echoes were observed. The septal leaflet of the tricuspid valve was lengthened and had a peculiar whiplike motion. Diagnostic findings represented inferior displacement of the septal leaflet on sagittal section and leftward displacement of the septal leaflet and its annulus on transverse section. These patients may also have striking right ventricular dilatation and true paradoxical septal motion. It is extremely difficult to appreciate these findings in any other mode than in the real-time studies.

TRICUSPID ATRESIA.—Tricuspid atresia is a severe form of congenital heart disease consisting of various degrees of hypoplasia of the right ventricle. The absence of any detectable tricuspid echo in either horizontal or sagittal cross section with an enlarged left ventricle and excessive mitral excursion allows this diagnosis to be made. This is a diagnosis of exclusion. Since more of the heart is seen with multicrystal echo, this lesion is more amenable to diagnosis by this technique than by single crystal study.[153] The transverse views in Position 2 are extremely useful as an aid to delineating the extent of the diminutive right ventricular cavity. Position 4 then should be used to assess the orientation of the great vessels, since transposition sometimes is seen in these patients.

Right Ventricular Outflow Tract Obstruction

The right ventricular outflow tract may be viewed adequately in Position 3 in 80% of children. This allows assessment of pulmonary artery contour. Infundibular or subvalvular right ventricular outflow tract obstruction is most difficult to assess, since apparent closing of the subvalvular region may be visualized if the transducer is not aligned directly along the course of the right ventricular outflow tract. Further, the definition obtained in this area makes it extremely difficult to obtain visualization of doming of the pulmonary valve or subtle areas of supravalvular pulmonary constriction. Nevertheless, some patients with valvular pulmonic stenosis have thickened immobile leaflets, and poststenotic dilatation sometimes may be observed (Fig. 7-14).

Left-to-Right Shunts

RIGHT VENTRICULAR VOLUME OVERLOAD.—Recent emphasis in the echocardiographic literature has been placed on abnormalities of septal motion in patients with right ventricular volume overload.[37,]

Fig. 7-14.—A Polaroid still (position 3) demonstrates poststenotic dilatation of the main pulmonary artery, distal to a stenotic pulmonary valve. The main pulmonary artery is labeled *MPA* just distal to the site of the valve cusp tissue, which is seen poorly.

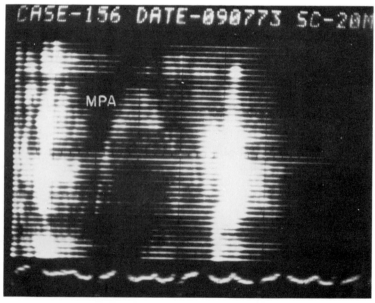

[125, 219] Normal and abnormal septal motion may easily be character-ized on the sagittal view of the heart obtained with the multicrystal echocardiographic system. In a study of 100 normals, the superior portion of the septum moved anteriorly during systole along with the aortic root.[99] A consistent finding was that the septum was hinged or pivoted at the junction of its upper one-third and lower two-thirds (Fig. 7-15). During systole, the lower two-thirds of the interventricular septum moves posteriorly, i.e., toward the anteriorly moving posteri-or left ventricular wall. This pivot point, which was located in the upper one-third of the septum in the 100 normal cases, was at the level of the mitral valve and explains the somewhat confusing pat-terns of septal motion that may be seen if echoes are obtained during single crystal study from the transition area in the anterior leaflet plane. Among 21 patients studied by the multicrystal echo system who had right ventricular volume overload, normal septal motion was observed in 6. True paradoxical septal motion, with the entire length of the septum moving anteriorly in systole, was observed in 8. Variable patterns with displacement of the hinge point inferiorly were observed in 7 patients. Ten of these 21 patients had atrial sep-tal defects. In 6 who had a pulmonary:systemic flow ratio of less than 2:1, all had normal septal motion, whereas 3 of 4 who had a pulmon-ary:systemic flow ratio greater than 2:1 had true paradoxical septal motion. Others in this group who had strikingly paradoxical septal motion included patients with Ebstein's anomaly and patients with significant pulmonary valvular insufficiency.[99] There are few false positives for paradoxical septal motion when over-all length of the ventricular septum is observed using two-dimensional, cross-sectional echocardiography.

VENTRICULAR SEPTAL DEFECT. — Unlike the experience reported by King et al.,[130] we have not routinely visualized ventricular septal defects with our technique and have experienced both false positives and many false negatives. Nevertheless, secondary signs of ventricu-lar septal defect may be helpful in establishing the diagnosis. These signs include increased left ventricular and atrial dimension and en-larged pulmonary artery.

Cyanotic Heart Disease

Diagnoses based on great vessel relations. The following varieties of cyanotic heart disease may be elucidated easily with cross-sectional echocardiography. The most important observations to be made in examining these patients include the relationship of the pos-terior great vessel and its semilunar valve to the mitral valve and

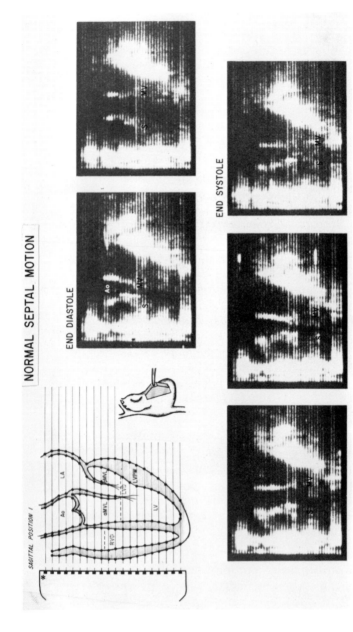

Fig. 7-15.—Normal septal motion as recorded in the sagittal plane by the multicrystal echocardiographic system is illustrated. The panel at top left is a schematic representation of the structures illustrated in the remaining five panels. At the beginning of systole, the anterior mitral valve leaflet (*MV*) moves posteriorly (right-hand panel—top). As left ventricular ejection proceeds, the inferior portion of the septum moves toward the posterior left ventricular wall and the superior portion of the septum moves anteriorly with the aortic root. *RVD* = right ventricular dimension; *Ao* = aorta; *aMVL, MV* = anterior mitral valve leaflet; *S* = septum; *LV* = left ventricle; *LVD* = left ventricular dimension; *pMVL* = posterior mitral valve leaflet; *LA* = left atrium; *LVPW* = left ventricular posterior wall. (By permission of the American Heart Association, Inc. Hagan, A. D., Francis, G., Sahn, D. J., Karliner, J., Friedman, W. F., and O'Rourke, R.: Ultrasound evaluation of systolic anterior septal motion in patients with and without right ventricular volume overload, Circulation 50:248, 1974.)

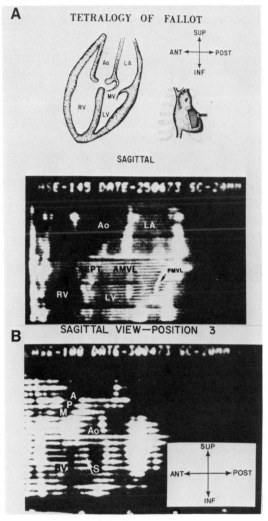

Fig. 7-16.—A, Position 1: Sagittal section in tetralogy of Fallot demonstrates aortic septal override, mitral aortic continuity and an enlarged right ventricle. The lower panel is a slightly retouched still frame selected from an 8-mm motion picture. *RV* = right ventricle; *SEPT* = septum; *LV* = left ventricle; *Ao* = aorta; *LA* = left atrium; *AMVL* = anterior mitral valve leaflet; *PMVL* = posterior mitral valve leaflet. **B,** Position 3, Sagittal: The normal posterior sweep of a small pulmonary artery in tetralogy of Fallot is illustrated in this still frame from an 8-mm motion picture. *MPA* = main pulmonary; *RV* = right ventricle; *S* = septum; *Ao* = aorta. (By permission of the American Heart Association, Inc. Sahn, D. J., Terry, R., O'Rourke, R., and Friedman, W. F.: Multiple crystal cross-sectional echocardiography in the diagnosis of cyanotic congenital heart disease, Circulation 50:230, 1974.)

septum, and great vessel orientation, as viewed in the second intercostal space, Transverse Position 4 (Fig. 7-5).

TETRALOGY OF FALLOT. — Major findings in tetralogy of Fallot are illustrated in Figure 7-16. The most important feature of this anomaly is observed in Sagittal Position 1 and corresponds to the single crystal echo observation of aortic-septal discontinuity.[28] As seen in Figure 7-16, A, there is a disruption of aortic septal continuity with preservation of mitral-aortic continuity. In this view, one can appreciate an enlarged ascending aorta that overrides the ventricular septum. Aortic override was visualized in 30 cyanotic children. Two of the 15 acyanotic patients had a clinical diagnosis of tetralogy of Fallot and had only minimal override. In a large group of acyanotic patients, those with extreme aortic root dilatation or marked right ventricular enlargement sometimes will seem to have override, but these represent false positives.[197] Additional tetralogy findings from views in Sagittal Position 1 include an increase in the cavity size of the right ventricle and a reduction in left atrial diameter unless a systemic artery – pulmonary artery shunt has been created.

Figure 7-16, B, shows that an assessment of the anatomy of the pulmonary artery can be made unless severe pulmonary hypoplasia exists. The pulmonary artery was identified in all of our patients, except for 2 who had pulmonary atresia and 1 who later was shown to have a Type 1 truncus arteriosus.

TRUNCUS ARTERIOSUS. — Findings of truncus arteriosus are quite similar to those described for tetralogy of Fallot. The main pulmonary artery cannot be identified in the usual location. Our patients have, in general, shown a marked degree of aortic septal override and often had multiple and unusual cusp echoes visualized within the truncal root. We would speculate that this latter finding reflects an abnormal number of cusps and, when present, may allow a distinction between patients with truncus arteriosus and other patients with pulmonary atresia and a ventricular septal defect ("pseudotruncus").

D-TRANSPOSITION OF THE GREAT VESSELS. — Major findings with situs solitis and D-transposition of the great vessels are illustrated in Figures 7-17 and 7-18. Single crystal descriptions of this anatomy have been attempts to define abnormal great vessel orientation.[27, 42, 128] (See also Chapter 4.) As viewed with cross-sectional echo, in Sagittal Position 1, the right ventricle is enlarged (Fig. 7-17, A). The aorta ascends retrosternally, in marked contrast to the posterior sweep of the normal pulmonary artery, which is found in this position in normals (Fig. 7-17, B). To visualize continuity between the anterior mi-

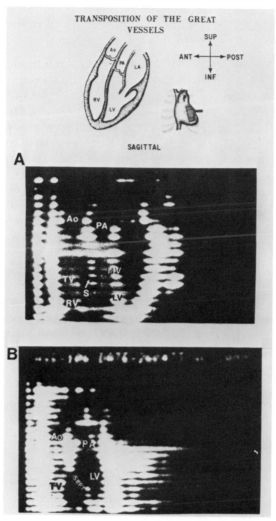

Fig. 7-17.—**A,** Position 1, Sagittal: Relationships of the great vessel in D-transposition are demonstrated in a still frame from an 8-mm motion picture. The aorta and pulmonary artery ascend one behind the other. *Ao* = aorta; *PA* = pulmonary artery; *TV* = tricuspid valve; *RV* = right ventricle; *S* = septum; *MV* = anterior mitral valve leaflet; *LV* = left ventricle. **B,** Position 1, Sagittal: The anteriorly placed aorta ascends retrosternally without a significant posterior sweep in this illustration from a patient with transposition of the great vessels. *TV* = tricuspid valve; *Ao* = aorta; *PA* = pulmonary artery; *SEPT* = septum; *LV* = left ventricle. (By permission of the American Heart Association, Inc. Sahn, D. J., Terry, R., O'Rourke, R., and Friedman, W. F.: Multiple crystal cross-sectional echocardiography in the diagnosis of cyanotic congenital heart disease, Circulation 50:230, 1974.)

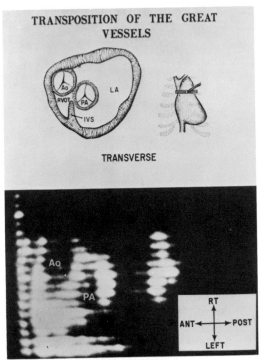

Fig. 7-18.—Position 4: D-transposition; the transverse section of transposed great vessels at the second intercostal space. Abnormal great vessel orientation is shown in this still frame from an 8-mm motion picture. The anteriorly placed vessel is to the right of the posteriorly placed vessel. Ao = aorta; PA = pulmonary artery; RVOT = right ventricular outflow tract; IVS = interventricular septum. (By permission of the American Heart Association, Inc. Sahn, D. J., Terry, R., O'Rourke, R., and Friedman, W. F.: Multiple crystal cross-sectional echocardiography in the diagnosis of cyanotic congenital heart disease, Circulation 50:230, 1974.)

tral leaflet and the semilunar valve of the posterior great vessel, it is necessary to angle the transducer leftward. Commonly, simultaneous sagittal plane visualization of the anterior and posterior great vessels shows one of the two ascending behind the other. The most important finding in our patients with D-transposition was observed in Transverse Position 4 (Fig. 7-18). In this view, the anterior great artery is to the right of the posterior great artery. Moreover, the course of the two great arteries in this plane may be traced to delineate their ventricle of origin. These maneuvers demonstrate that the anterior rightward vessel (aorta) originates from the right ventricle whereas the posterior leftward vessel (pulmonary artery) originates from the left ventricle. We recognize that rare forms of transposition may demonstrate unusual great vessel orientation. In the absence of dextrocardia, however, in our own series, we saw no other situation in which the anterior vessel was to the right.

DOUBLE OUTLET RIGHT VENTRICLE. — In 2 patients with double outlet right ventricle of the Taussig-Bing type there was abnormal great vessel orientation. The aorta was anterior and to the right, but the great vessels were essentially side by side. Both semilunar valves were in the same superior-inferior plane. Further, the posterior great vessel was displaced anteriorly from the mitral annulus so that there was mitral pulmonic discontinuity.[25, 100, 170, 171] As a subpulmonary conus existed between the mitral annulus and the semilunar

Fig. 7-19. — Position 1, Sagittal: This Polaroid still frame demonstrates the relationships of the aorta and the pulmonary artery in a patient with single ventricle transposition and pulmonic stenosis. The ascending aorta is markedly dilated. The valvular structure within the single ventricle is not well defined, but no septation is visible. Ao = aorta; MPA = main pulmonary artery; SV = single ventricle. (By permission of the American Heart Association, Inc. Sahn, D. J., Terry, R., O'Rourke, R., and Friedman, W. F.: Multiple crystal cross-sectional echocardiography in the diagnosis of cyanotic congenital heart disease, Circulation 50:230, 1974.)

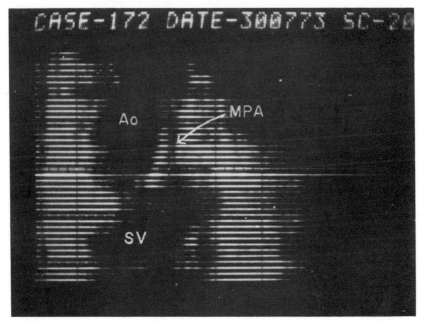

valve of the posterior vessel, the superior-inferior relationships of the posterior, semilunar and AV valves likewise were abnormal. As such, there was mitral pulmonic discontinuity in both the anterior and posterior as well as in the superior-inferior relationships.

SINGLE VENTRICLE. — This rare and complex form of congenital heart disease consists of single or double inlet ventricle. This is the most common form of single ventricle. Most of these patients have transposition of the great vessels. The anatomy is extremely complex and yet a good over-all view of the abnormality is characterized by the absence of the septal echo. One or two atrioventricular valves empty into the large cavity. In this case, the anterior vessel (aorta) originates from a small outflow chamber and is markedly dilated and

Fig. 7-20. — Position 2: Transverse section in a patient with L-transposition of the great vessels shows displaced side-by-side ventricles and AV valves. The interventricular septum lies in a plane parallel to incident sound waves and is not visualized. *MV* = right-sided mitral valve; *TV* = left-sided tricuspid valve; *LA* = left atrium; *RA* = right atrium; *RIGHT-SIDED VENT.* = right-sided morphologic left ventricle; *LEFT-SIDED VENT.* = left-sided morphologic right ventricle. (By permission of the American Heart Association, Inc. Sahn, D. J., Terry, R., O'Rourke, R., and Friedman, W. F.: Multiple crystal cross-sectional echocardiography in the diagnosis of cyanotic congenital heart disease, Circulation 50:230, 1974.)

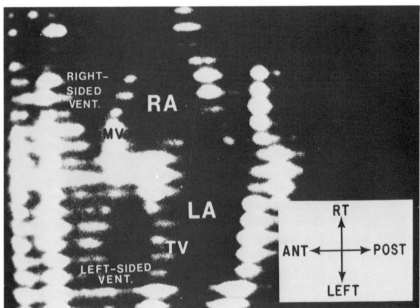

tortuous. As usual, there was subpulmonic and pulmonary outflow tract obstruction with a rather small posteriorly placed pulmonary artery (Fig. 7-19).

L-transposition

In Transverse Position 4 in patients with L-transposition, the great vessel orientation appears to be normal, with the anterior vessel (now the aorta) located to the left; however, a correct diagnosis may be made by tracing both vessels back to their ventricles of origin. The anterior leftward great artery arises from the anterior leftward portion of the left-sided ventricle and is not in continuity with the left-sided AV valve. Further, Sagittal Position 1 of the anterior vessel shows it to have a long retrosternal sweep characteristic of the aorta in transposition anomalies. In Transverse Position 2, both ventricles and their atrioventricular valves appear to lie side by side (Fig. 7-20). The ventricular septum, like the atrial septum, is on a straight anteroposterior plane parallel to incident sound waves and therefore is not visualized.

GENERAL REMARKS

1. In the absence of successful definition of the specific structural abnormality characteristic of one of the above lesions, multiscan echocardiography still may be useful in the evaluation of congenital heart disease, since it is a reliable approach to the measurement of ventricular dimension and may allow the assembly of a physiologic picture of chamber or great vessel enlargement.[20]

2. The M-mode echocardiograms obtained from single crystals within the format allow obtaining precise dimensional data with precise spatial orientation.

3. All four multicrystal cross-sectional echocardiographic positions may be appropriately modified to the right sternal border in patients with dextrocardia. The technique provides ease of identification of the various structures in real-time motion.

4. The reliability of spatial orientation aids in the reproducibility of this examination and allows serial assessments of valve motion, great vessel and chamber size, as well as of the progression of post-stenotic dilatation or valvular obstruction in patients as they grow. The technique has great promise for the noninvasive diagnosis and serial follow-up of patients with congenital heart disease.

Postscript

AT THE END OF THIS BOOK and for the future, several comments are in order.

While this book is being read, many parts are already outdated. It is only as current as the submission date, June 1974.

In addition to echocardiography, we learned much about illustration. For example, it was necessary to avoid long strips, for photography reduced the figure size too much. In most instances, we were more successful if we made one point at a time with an echocardiogram. We tried to include enough echo material to allow others to evaluate it critically. The paper cutter and double-backed tape mounting technique were used throughout. Labeling original echoes was done with a polyethylene carbon ribbon typewriter. These did not "bleed" into the paper. Rub-on transfer type letters were used for labeling glossy photographs because typing does not imprint the photograph effectively.

We did not retouch echoes. Enough troubles with interpretation occur without altering the original.

Nearly all the echoes in the book were recorded on Honeywell light-sensitive paper. Photographic representation of the Honeywell strips was very poor at first. A discussion of the technique follows.

Finally, we realized normal values were important; this was brought home so clearly when we evaluated echoes of children with different forms of congenital heart disease. Subtle deviations from fifth and ninety-fifth percentiles are exquisitely sensitive in correlating with the pathology. Evaluation of echoes in this manner and development of more normal data and elucidation of normal variation should be accomplished during the next few years.

And now, back to the ground.

Echocardiography Photographic Technique

THE ORIGINAL CONTRAST of an echocardiogram has very limited tonal value. Most are brown tracings on brown paper and do not photograph well with ultra high contrast film. Therefore, the following method was developed for reproducing high-quality echocardiograms for publication and black and white slides for teaching as done by the Medical Photography Department of the Medical Audiovisual Services.

Lighting — Four 150-watt floods set at a 45° angle to the original tracing. The lights are attached to a Colortran Colortru Converter and boosted to 3200^k.

Film — 135-mm High Contrast Copy film, prepackaged, ASA 64.

Exposure — With four lights at 3200^k, the exposure is 1 second at f/11.

Development — Kodak D76 straight for 6 minutes at 68° F.

Printing (Slides) — Fine Grain Positive Kodak film 7302. Exposed for ¾ second on a contact printer and developed in Dektol 1:2 until desired contrast is reached.

Prints — Ektamatic SC "F" paper using Ektamatic stabilizer. Filter is a #3 polycontrast filter and exposure time is 6 seconds at f/11. Prints are fixed and washed after development.

CLIFF POLLACK

CHIEF MEDICAL PHOTOGRAPHER
MEDICAL AUDIOVISUAL SERVICES
ARIZONA MEDICAL CENTER

REFERENCES

1. Abbasi, A. S., Eber, L. M., MacAlpin, R. N., and Kattus, A. A.: Ventricular septal asynergy in complete left bundle branch block, Circulation 48(Supp. IV): 135, 1973.
2. Abbasi, A. S., MacAlpin, R. N., Eber, L. M., and Pearce, M. L.: Echocardiographic diagnosis of idiopathic hypertrophic cardiomyopathy without outflow obstruction, Circulation 46:897, 1972.
3. Abbasi, A. S., MacAlpin, R. N., Eber, L. M., and Pearce, M. L.: Left ventricular hypertrophy diagnosed by echocardiography, N. Engl. J. Med. 289:118, 1973.
4. Abbasi, A. S., MacAlpin, R. N., Eber, L. M., and Pearce, M. L.: The diagnosis of primary and secondary left ventricular hypertrophy by echocardiography, Circulation 46(Supp. II): 62, 1972.
5. Alderman, E. L., Rytand, D. A., Crow, R. S., Finegan, R. E., and Harrison, D. C.: Normal and prosthetic atrioventricular valve motion in atrial flutter. Correlation of ultrasound, vectorcardiographic, and phonocardiographic findings, Circulation 45:1206, 1972.
6. Allen, H. D., Blieden, L. C., Stone, F. M., Bessinger, F. B., and Lucas, R. V.: Echocardiographic demonstration of a right ventricular tumor in a neonate, J. Pediatr. 84:854, 1974.
7. Askanas, A., Rajszys, R., Sadowski, Z., and Stopczyk, M.: Measurement of the thickness of the left ventricular wall in man using the ultrasound technique, Pol. Med. J. 9:62, 1970.
8. Baron, M. G.: Abnormalities of the mitral valve in endocardial cushion defects, Circulation 45:672, 1972.
9. Basford, J., Kamigaki, M., Clark, R., Taylor, B., and Cohn, K.: The use of echocardiography in distinguishing different varieties of mitral regurgitation, Circulation 46(Supp. II):41, 1972.
10. Belenkie, I., Nutter, D., Clark, D., McCraw, B., and Raizner, A. E.: Assessment of left ventricular dimensions and function by echocardiography, Am. J. Cardiol. 31:755, 1973.
11. Betriu, A., Wigle, E. D., Felderhof, D. H., and McLouglin, M. J.: Prolapse of the posterior leaflet of the mitral valve associated with secundum atrial septal defect, Am. J. Cardiol. 33:126, 1974.
12. Blieden, L. C., Castañeda, A. R., Nicoloff, D. M., Lillehei, C. W., and Moller, J. H.: Prosthetic valve replacement in children. Results in 44 patients, Ann. Thorac. Surg. 14:545, 1972.
13. Bolton, M. R., King, J. F., Reis, R. L., Pugh, D. M., Polumbo, R. A., Dunn, M. I., and Mason, D. T.: Alterations of echocardiographic features of IHSS by operation. Simultaneous comparison with pre, early and late postoperative catheterizations in the same patients undergoing ventricular septal myectomy, Circulation 48(Supp. IV):47, 1973.
14. Bom, N.: New Concepts in Echocardiography (Leiden: Stenfert-Kroese, N.V., 1971).
15. Bom, N., Lancée, C. T. Honkoop, J., and Hugenholtz, P. G.: Ultrasonic viewer for cross-sectional analyses of moving cardiac structures, Biomed. Eng. 6:500, 1971.
16. Bom, N., Lancée, C. T., van Zweiten, G., Kloster, F. E., and Roelandt,

J.: Multiscan echocardiography. Technical description, Circulation 48: 1066, 1973.

17. Brown, O. R., Harrison, D. C., and Popp, R. L.: Echocardiographic study of right ventricular hypertension producing asymmetric septal hypertrophy, Circulation 48(Supp. IV):47, 1973.

18. Cahill, N. S., Lipp, H., Gambetta, M., Al-Sadir, J., King, S., and Resnekov, L.: Assessment of left ventricular function in acute myocardial infarction by echocardiography, Circulation 46(Supp. II):136, 1972.

19. Carter, W. H., and Bowman, C. R.: Estimation of shunt flow in isolated ventricular septal defect by echocardiogram, Circulation 48(Supp. IV): 64, 1973.

20. ten Cate, F. J., Kloster, F. E., Roelandt, J., van Dorp, W. G., and Hugenholtz, P. G.: Cardiac dimensions by multiple element echocardiography, Circulation 48(Supp. IV):223, 1973.

21. Chandraratna, P. A. N., Nanda, N. C., Shah, P. M., Hodges, M., and Gramiak, R.: Echocardiographic study of left atrial size in acute myocardial infarction, Circulation 46(Supp. II):138, 1972.

22. Chang, S., and Feigenbaum, H.: Subxiphoid echocardiography, J. Clin. Ultrasound 1:14, 1973.

23. Chesler, E., Joffe, H. S., Vecht, R., Beck, W., and Schrire, V.: Ultrasound cardiography in single ventricle and the hypoplastic left and right heart syndromes, Circulation 42:123, 1970.

24. Chesler, E., Joffe, H. S., Beck, W., and Schrire, V.: Echocardiography in the diagnosis of congenital heart disease, Pediatr. Clin. North Am. 18: 1163, 1971.

25. Chesler, E., Joffe, H. S., Beck, W., and Schrire, V.: Echocardiographic recognition of mitral-semilunar valve discontinuity, Circulation 43:725, 1971.

26. Chung, K., Alexson, C. G., Manning, J. A., and Gramiak, R.: Echocardiography in truncus arteriosus: The value of pulmonic valve detection, Circulation 48:281, 1973.

27. Chung, K. J., Gramiak, R., Nanda, N. C., and Manning, J.: Echocardiographic diagnosis of transposition of the great vessels, Circulation 46(Supp. II):38, 1972.

28. Chung, K. J., Nanda, N. C., Manning, J. A., and Gramiak, R.: Echocardiographic findings in tetralogy of Fallot, Am. J. Cardiol. 31:126, 1973.

29. Clark, C. E., Henry, W. L., and Epstein, S. E.: The sensitivity and specificity of echocardiography in diagnosing IHSS by detection of asymmetrical septal hypertrophy, Circulation 46(Supp. II):139, 1972.

30. Cooper, R. H., O'Rourke, R. A., Karliner, J. S., Peterson, K. L., and Leopold, G. R.: Comparison of ultrasound and cineangiographic measurements of the mean rate of circumferential fiber shortening in man, Circulation 46:914, 1972.

31. Corya, B. C., Feigenbaum, H., Rasmussen, S., and Black, M.: Echocardiographic examination of the anterior left ventricular wall in patients with coronary artery disease, Am. J. Cardiol. 33:132, 1974.

32. Crews, T. L., Pridie, R. B., Benham, R., and Leatham, A.: Auscultatory and phonocardiographic findings in Ebstein's anomaly. Correlation of first heart sound with ultrasonic records of tricuspid valve movement, Br. Heart J. 34:681, 1972.

33. Danford, H. G., Danford, D. A., Mielke, J. E., and Peterson, L. F.: Echocardiographic evaluation of the hemodynamic effects of chronic aortic insufficiency with observations on left ventricular performance, Circulation 48:253, 1973.
34. Davis, R. H., Feigenbaum, H., Chang, S., Konecke, L., and Dillon, J. C.: Echocardiographic manifestations of discrete subaortic stenosis, Am. J. Cardiol. 33:277, 1974.
35. DeMaria, A., King, J. F., Bonanno, J. A., Lies, J. E., Massumi, R. A., Amsterdam, E. A., and Mason, D. T.: Effects of electroversion of atrial fibrillation on cardiac function. Echographic assessment of atrial transport, mitral movement and ventricular performance, Circulation 48 (Supp. IV):158, 1973.
36. DeMaria, A., King, J. F., Bogren, H., Bonanno, J. A., Massumi, R. A., Zelis, R., and Mason, D. T.: The variable spectrum of echocardiographic manifestations of mitral valve prolapse, Circulation 48(Supp. IV):63, 1973.
37. Diamond, M. A., Dillon, J. C., Haine, C. L., Chang, S., and Feigenbaum, H.: Echocardiographic features of atrial septal defect, Circulation 43:129, 1971.
38. Dillon, J. C., Chang, S., and Feigenbaum, H.: Echocardiographic manifestations of left bundle branch block, Circulation 48(Supp. IV):126, 1973.
39. Dillon, J. C., Chang, S., and Feigenbaum, H.: Echocardiographic manifestations of left bundle branch block, Circulation 49:876, 1974.
40. Dillon, J. C., Haine, C. L., Chang, S., and Feigenbaum, H.: Use of echocardiography in patients with prolapsed mitral valve, Circulation 43:503, 1971.
41. Dillon, J. C., Feigenbaum, H., Konecke, L. L., Davis, R. H., and Chang, S.: Echocardiographic manifestations of valvular vegetations, Am. Heart J. 86:698, 1973.
42. Dillon, J. C., Feigenbaum, H., Konecke, L. L., Keutel, J., Hurwitz, R. A., Davis, R. H., and Chang, S.: Echocardiographic manifestations of d-transposition of the great vessels, Am. J. Cardiol. 32:74, 1973.
43. Dippel, W. F., and Kerber, R. E.: Mechanism of the echocardiographic abnormality of interventricular septum motion in right ventricular volume overload, Circulation 46(Supp. II):36, 1972.
44. Duchak, J. M., Jr., Chang, S., and Feigenbaum, H.: Echocardiographic features of torn chordae tendineae, Am. J. Cardiol. 29:260, 1972.
45. Duchak, J., Chang, S., and Feigenbaum, H.: The posterior mitral valve echo and the echocardiographic diagnosis of mitral stenosis, Am. J. Cardiol. 29:628, 1972.
46. Edler, I., et al.: Ultrasound cardiography, Acta Med. Scand., Supplement 370, 1961.
47. Edler, I.: The diagnostic use of ultrasound in heart disease, Acta Med. Scand. 308:32, 1955.
48. Edler, I.: Ultrasound cardiography in mitral valve stenosis, Am. J. Cardiol. 19:18, 1967.
49. Effert, S., and Domanig, E.: The diagnosis of intra-atrial tumor and thrombi by the ultrasonic echo method, Ger. Med. Mon. 4:1, 1959.
50. Effert, S., Erkens, H., and Grossebrockhoff, F.: Ultrasonic echo method in cardiological diagnosis, Ger. Med. Mon. 2:325, 1957.

51. Effert, S.: Pre- and postoperative evaluation of mitral stenosis by ultrasound, Am. J. Cardiol. 19:59, 1967.
52. Ellis, K., and King, D. L.: Pericarditis and pericardial effusion, Radiol. Clin. North Am. 11:393, 1973.
53. Enos, W. F., Jr., Holmes, R. H., and Beyer, J. C.: Coronary artery disease in American soldiers killed in Korea, JAMA 152:1090, 1953.
54. Eshaghpour, E., Turnoff, H. B., Kingsley, B., and Linhart, J. W.: Echocardiographic features of endocardial cushion defect, Am. J. Cardiol. 33:135, 1974.
55. Feigenbaum, H.: Echocardiographic diagnosis of pericardial effusion, Am. J. Cardiol. 26:475, 1970.
56. Feigenbaum, H.: Echocardiography (Philadelphia: Lea & Febiger, 1972).
57. Feigenbaum, H., Linback, R. E., and Nasser, W. K.: Hemodynamic studies before and after instrumental mitral commissurotomy. A reappraisal of the patho-physiology of mitral stenosis and the efficacy of mitral valvotomy, Circulation 38:261, 1968.
58. Feigenbaum, H., Popp, R. L., Chip, J. N., and Haine, C. L.: Left ventricular wall thickness measured by ultrasound, Arch. Intern. Med. 121:391, 1968.
59. Feigenbaum, H., Popp, R. L., Wolfe, S. B., Troy, B. L., Pombo, J. F., Haine, C. L., and Dodge, H. T.: Ultrasound measurements of the left ventricle. A correlative study with angiocardiography, Arch. Intern. Med. 129:461, 1972.
60. Feigenbaum, H., Stone, J. M., Lee, D. A., Nasser, W. K., and Chang, S.: Identification of ultrasound echoes from the left ventricle by use of intracardiac injections of indocyanine green, Circulation 51:615, 1970.
61. Feigenbaum, H., Waldhausen, J. A., and Hyde, L. P.: Ultrasound diagnosis of pericardial effusion, JAMA 191:107, 1965.
62. Feigenbaum, H., Zaky, A., and Grabhorn, L. L.: Cardiac motion in patients with pericardial effusion, Circulation 34:611, 1966.
63. Feigenbaum, H., Zaky, A., and Waldhausen, J. A.: Use of reflected ultrasound in detecting pericardial effusion, Am. J. Cardiol. 19:84, 1967.
64. Feigenbaum, H., Zaky, A., and Waldhausen, J. A.: Use of ultrasound in the diagnosis of pericardial effusion, Ann. Intern. Med. 65:443, 1966.
65. Feizi, O., Symons, C., and Yacoub, M.: Echocardiography of normal and diseased aortic valve. Proceedings British Cardiac Society, Br. Heart J. 35:560, 1973.
66. Finegan, R. E., and Harrison, D. C.: Diagnosis of left atrial myxoma by echocardiography, N. Engl. J. Med. 282:1022, 1970.
67. Fogelman, A. M., Abbasi, A. S., Pearce, M. L., and Kattus, A. A.: Echocardiographic abnormalities of the posterior left ventricular wall during angina pectoris, Circulation 46(Supp. II): 42, 1972.
68. Fogelman, A. M., Abbasi, A. S., Pearce, M. L., and Kattus, A. A.: Echocardiographic study of the abnormal motion of the posterior left ventricular wall during angina pectoris, Circulation 46:905, 1972.
69. Fortuin, N. J., and Craige, E.: On the mechanism of Austin Flint murmur, Circulation 45:558, 1972.
70. Fortuin, N. J., Hood, W. P., and Craige, E.: Evaluation of left ventricular function by echocardiography, Circulation 46:26, 1972.
71. Fortuin, N. J., Hood, W. P., Jr., Sherman, M. E., and Craige, E.: Deter-

mination of left ventricular volumes by ultrasound, Circulation 44:575, 1971.

72. Gabor, G. E., Winsberg, F., and Bloom, H. S.: Electrical and mechanical alternation in pericardial effusion, Chest 59:341, 1971.

73. Gasul, B. M., Arcilla, R. A., and Lev, M.: *Heart Disease in Children* (Philadelphia and Montreal: J. B. Lippincott Company, 1966).

74. Gibson, D. G., and Brown, D.: Measurement of instantaneous left ventricular volumes and filling rate in man by echocardiography, Br. Heart J. 35:559, 1973.

75. Gibson, T. C., Starek, P. J. K., Moos, S., and Craige, E.: Echocardiographic and phonocardiographic characteristics of the Lillehei-Kaster mitral valve prosthesis, Circulation 49:434, 1974.

76. Gimenez, J. L., Winters, W. L., Jr., Davila, J. C., Connel, J., and Klein, K. S.: Dynamics of the Starr-Edwards ball valve prosthesis; a cinefluorographic and ultrasonic study in humans, Am. J. Med. Sci. 250:652, 1965.

77. Glaser, J.: Echocardiographic studies of mitral valve. Letter to the editor, Am. Heart J. 85:847, 1973.

78. Glaser, J., Bharati, S., Whitman, V., and Liebman, J.: Echocardiographic findings in patients with anomalous origin of the left coronary artery, Circulation 48(Supp. IV):63, 1973.

79. Glaser, J., Whitman, V., and Liebman, J.: The differential diagnosis of total anomalous pulmonary venous drainage in infancy by echocardiography, Circulation 46(Supp. II):38, 1972.

80. Glasser, S. P., *et al.*: Left atrial myxoma, Am. J. Med. 50:113, 1971.

81. Goldberg, B. B.: Suprasternal ultrasonography, JAMA 15:245, 1971.

82. Goldberg, B. B., Ostrum, B. J., and Isard, H. J.: Ultrasonic determination of pericardial effusion, JAMA 202:927, 1967.

83. Goldman, D. E., and Hueter, T. F.: Tabular data of the velocity and absorption of high-frequency sound in mammalian tissue, J. Acoust. Soc. Am. 28:35, 1956.

84. Goldschlager, A., Popper, R., Goldschlager, N., Gerbode, F., and Prozan, G.: Right atrial myxoma with right to left shunt and polycythemia presenting as congenital heart disease, Am. J. Cardiol. 30:82, 1972.

85. Goodman, D. J., Harrison, D. C., and Popp, R. L.: Echocardiographic features of primary pulmonary hypertension, Circulation 48(Supp. IV):170, 1973.

86. Gordon, D.: *Ultrasound as a Diagnostic and Surgical Tool* (Baltimore: The Williams & Wilkins Company, 1964).

87. Gramiak, R., Chung, K. J., Nanda, N., and Manning, J.: Echocardiographic diagnosis of transposition of the great vessels, Radiology 106:187, 1973.

88. Gramiak, R., and Nanda, N. C.: Echocardiographic diagnosis of ostium primum septal defect, Circulation 46(Supp. II):37, 1972.

89. Gramiak, R., Nanda, N. C., and Shah, P. M.: Echocardiographic detection of the pulmonary valve, Radiology 102:153, 1972.

90. Gramiak, R., and Shah, P. M.: Echocardiography of the normal and diseased aortic valve, Radiology 96:1, 1970.

91. Gramiak, R., and Shah, P. M.: Cardiac ultrasonography: A review of current applications, Radiol. Clin. North Am. 9:469, 1971.

92. Gramiak, R., Shah, P. M., and Kramer, D. H.: Ultrasound cardiography: Contrast studies in anatomy and function, Radiology 92:939, 1969.

93. Griffith, J. M., Henry, W. L., and Epstein, S. E.: Real time two-dimensional echocardiography, Circulation 48(Supp. IV):124, 1973.

94. Grossman, W., McLaurin, L. P., Moos, S. P., Stefadouros, M., and Young, D. T.: Wall thickness and diastolic properties of the left ventricle, Circulation 49:129, 1974.

95. Guntheroth, W. G.: Pediatric Electrocardiography—Normal and Abnormal Patterns, Incorporating the Vector Approach (Philadelphia: W. B. Saunders Company, 1965).

96. Gustafson, A.: Correlation between ultrasound cardiography, hemodynamics and surgical findings in mitral stenosis, Am. J. Cardiol. 19:32, 1967.

97. Hagan, A. D., Deely, W. J., Sahn, D. J., and Friedman, W. F.: Echocardiographic criteria for normal newborn infants, Circulation 48:1221, 1973.

98. Hagan, A., Francis, G., Sahn, D., Karliner, J., Friedman, W., and O'Rourke, R.: Systolic anterior septal motion—an unreliable echocardiographic finding, Circulation 48(Supp. IV):173, 1973.

99. Hagan, A. D., Francis, G., Sahn, D. J., Karliner, J., Friedman, W. F., and O'Rourke, R.: Ultrasound evaluation of systolic anterior septal motion in patients with and without right ventricular volume overload, Circulation 50:248, 1974.

100. Hallermann, F. J., Kincaid, O. W., Ritter, D. G., and Titus, J. L.: Mitral-semilunar valve relationships in the angiography of cardiac malformations, Radiology 94:63, 1970.

101. Henry, W. L., Clark, C. E., and Epstein, S. E.: Asymmetric septal hypertrophy, Circulation 47:225, 1973.

102. Henry, W. L., Clark, C. E., Glancy, D. L., and Epstein, S. E.: Echocardiographic measurement of the left ventricular outflow gradient in idiopathic hypertrophic subaortic stenosis, N. Engl. J. Med. 288:989, 1973.

103. Henry, W. L., Maron, B. J., Griffith, J. M., and Epstein, S. E.: The differential diagnosis of anomalies of the great vessels by real-time, two-dimensional echocardiography, Am. J. Cardiol. 33:143, 1974.

104. Hertz, C. H.: Ultrasonic engineering in heart diagnosis, Am. J. Cardiol. 19:6, 1967.

105. Hirata, T., Wolfe, S. B., Popp, R. L., Helmen, C. H., and Feigenbaum, H.: Estimation of left atrial size using ultrasound, Am. Heart J. 78:43, 1969.

106. Hirschfeld, S., Meyer, R. A., and Kaplan, S.: Non-invasive right and left systolic time intervals by echocardiography, Pediatr. Res. 8:350, 1974.

107. Horowitz, M. S., et al.: Reliability and sensitivity of echocardiography in pericardial effusion, Circulation 48(Supp. IV):125, 1973.

108. Inoue, K., Smulyan, H., Mookherjee, S., and Eich, R. H.: Ultrasonic measurement of left ventricular wall motion in acute myocardial infarction, Circulation 43:778, 1971.

109. Jacobs, J. J., Feigenbaum, H., Corya, B. C., Haine, C. L., Black, M., and Chang, S.: Echocardiographic detection of left ventricular asynergy, Circulation 46(Supp. II):42, 1972.

110. Jacobs, J. J., Feigenbaum, H., Corya, B. C., and Phillips, J. F.: Detection of left ventricular asynergy by echocardiography, Circulation 48: 263, 1973.
111. Johnson, M. L., Holmes, J. H., and Paton, B. C.: Echocardiographic determination of mitral disc valve excursion, Circulation 47:1274, 1973.
112. Johnson, M. L., Holmes, J. H., Spangler, R. D., and Paton, B. C.: Usefulness of echocardiography in patients undergoing mitral valve surgery, J. Thorac. Cardiovasc. Surg. 64:922, 1972.
113. Johnson, M. L., Kisslo, J., Habersberger, P. G., and Wallace, A. G.: Echocardiographic evaluation of aortic valvular disease, Circulation 48 (Supp. IV):46, 1973.
114. Johnson, M. L., Paton, B. C., and Holmes, J. H.: Ultrasonic evaluation of prosthetic valve motion, Circulation 41(Supp. II):3, 1970.
115. Johnson, S. L., Baker, D. W., Lute, R. A., and Kawabori, I.: Detection of left-to-right shunts and right ventricular outflow tract obstruction by Doppler echocardiography, Circulation 48(Supp. IV):82, 1973.
116. Johnson, S. L., Baker, D. W., Lute, R. A., and Murray, J. A.: Detection of mitral regurgitation by Doppler echocardiography, Am. J. Cardiol. 33:147, 1974.
117. Joyner, C. R., Dyrda, I., and Reid, J. M.: Behavior of the anterior leaflet of the mitral valve in patients with the Austin Flint murmur, Clin. Res. 14:251, 1966.
118. Joyner, C. R., Hey, E. D., Johnson, J., and Reid, J. M.: Reflected ultrasound in the diagnosis of tricuspid stenosis, Am. J. Cardiol. 19:66, 1967.
119. Joyner, C. R., and Reid, J. M.: Application of ultrasound in cardiology and cardiovascular physiology, Prog. Cardiovasc. Dis. 5:482, 1963.
120. Kamigaki, M., and Goldschlager, N.: Echocardiographic analysis of mitral valve motion in atrial septal defect, Am. J. Cardiol. 30:343, 1972.
121. Karliner, J., Ludbrook, P., O'Rourke, R., Peterson, K., and Leopold, G.: Posterior wall velocity—an unreliable index of left ventricular contractility, Circulation 46(Supp. II):45, 1972.
122. Keith, J. D., Rowe, R. D., and Vlad, P.: *Heart Disease in Infancy and Childhood* (New York: The Macmillan Company, 1967).
123. Kelly, E.: *Ultrasonic Energy; Biological Investigations and Medical Applications* (Urbana: University of Illinois Press, 1965).
124. Kerber, R. E.: Echocardiographic detection of regional myocardial infarction, Circulation 46(Supp. II):42, 1972.
125. Kerber, R. E., Dippel, W. F., and Abboud, F. M.: Abnormal motion of the interventricular septum in right ventricular volume overload, Circulation 48:86, 1973.
126. Kerber, R. E., Isaeff, D. M., and Hancock, E. W.: Echocardiographic patterns in patients with the syndrome of systolic click and late systolic murmur, N. Engl. J. Med. 284:691, 1971.
127. Kim, H., *et al.*: An attempt to correlate the mitral valve echogram with the hemodynamics of patients with pure mitral insufficiency, Jap. Circ. J. 37:393, 1973.
128. King, D. L., Steeg, C. N., and Ellis, K.: Demonstrations of transposition of the great arteries by cardiac ultrasonography, Radiology 107:181, 1973.
129. King, D. L.: Cardiac ultrasonography—cross-sectional ultrasonic imaging of the heart, Circulation 47:843, 1973.

130. King, D. L., Steeg, C., and Ellis, K.: Visualization of ventricular septal defects by cardiac ultrasonography, Circulation 48:1215, 1973.
131. King, J. F., DeMaria, A. N., Bonanno, J. A., and Mason, D. T.: The temporal sequence of myocardial contraction in the bundle branch block determined by echocardiography, Circulation 48(Supp. IV):127, 1973.
132. Kingsley, B.: Stroke volume and cardiac output by echocardiography, J. Audio Eng. Soc. 18:692, 1970.
133. Kisslo, J. A., Wolfson, S., Hammond, G. L., and Cohen, L. S.: Echocardiography in the assessment of left ventricular function after saphenous vein bypass, Circulation 46(Supp. II):68, 1972.
134. Klein, J. J., and Segal, B. L.: Pericardial effusion diagnosed by reflected ultrasound, Am. J. Cardiol. 22:57, 1968.
135. Kloster, F. E., Roelandt, J., ten Cate, F. J., Bom, N., and Hugenholtz, P. G.: Multiscan echocardiography. Technique and initial clinical results, Circulation 48:1075, 1973.
136. Kortis, J. B., and Moghadam, A. N.: Echocardiographic diagnosis of left atrial myxoma, Chest 58:550, 1970.
137. Kossoff, G.: Diagnostic applications of ultrasound in cardiology, Australas. Radiol. 10:101, 1966.
138. Kotler, M. N.: Tricuspid valve in Ebstein's anomaly, Circulation 47:597, 1973.
139. Levy, A. M., Leaman, D. M., and Hanson, J. S.: Effects of digoxin on systolic time intervals of neonates and infants, Circulation 46:816, 1972.
140. Lies, J. E., Bonanno, J. A., DeMaria, A., and Mason, D. T.: Echographic detection of subclinical cardiomyopathy, Circulation 48(Supp. IV):192, 1973.
141. Lundström, N. R.: Echocardiography in the diagnosis of Ebstein's anomaly of the tricuspid valve, Circulation 47:597, 1973.
142. Lundström, N. R.: Echocardiography in the diagnosis of congenital mitral stenosis and in evaluation of the results of mitral valvotomy, Radiology 106:238, 1973.
143. Lundström, N. R.: Ultrasound cardiographic studies of the mitral valve region in young infants with mitral atresia, mitral stenosis, hypoplasia of the left ventricle, and cor triatriatum, Circulation 45:324, 1972.
144. Lundström, N. R.: Echocardiography in the diagnosis of congenital mitral stenosis and in evaluation of the results of mitral valvotomy, Circulation 46:44, 1972.
145. Lundström, N. R., and Edler, I.: Ultrasound cardiography in infants and children, Acta Paediatr. Scand. 60:117, 1971.
146. Mahringer, W., and Hausen, W. J.: The origin of the ultrasound echocardiogram in mitral stenosis. Studies on prosthetic valves with the aid of roentgen cinematography, Z. Kreislaufforsch. 58:1193, 1969.
147. Mahringer, W., and Hausen, W. J.: Ultrasound cardiogram in patients with mitral valve disc prostheses, Angiology 21:336, 1970.
148. Martinez, E. C., Giles, T. D., and Burch, G. E.: Echocardiographic diagnosis of left atrial myxoma, Am. J. Cardiol. 33:281, 1974.
149. McCann, W. D., Harbold, N. B., and Giuliani, E. R.: The echocardiogram in right ventricular overload, JAMA 221:1243, 1972.
150. McDonald, I. G.: Echocardiographic demonstration of abnormal motion

of the interventricular septum in left bundle branch block, Circulation 48:272, 1973.

151. McDonald, I. G., Feigenbaum, H., and Chang, S.: Analysis of left ventricular wall motion by reflected ultrasound, Circulation 46:14, 1972.

152. McDonald, I. G., Feigenbaum, H., and Chang, S.: Analysis of left ventricular wall motion by reflected ultrasound. Application to assessment of myocardial function, Radiology 106:238, 1973.

153. Meyer, R. A., and Kaplan, S.: Echocardiography in the diagnosis of hypoplasia of the left or right ventricles in the neonate, Circulation 46: 55, 1972.

154. Meyer, R. A., and Kaplan, S.: Radionuclide pericardial scan. Is it outmoded by echocardiography?, Pediatrics 49:637, 1972.

155. Meyer, R., Schwartz, D. C., Benzing, G., and Kaplan, S.: Ventricular septum in right ventricular volume overload, Am. J. Cardiol. 30:349, 1972.

156. Meyer, R. A., Stockert, J., and Kaplan, S.: Echographic determination of left ventricular volumes, Pediatr. Res. 7:300, 1973.

157. Millward, D. K., McLaurin, L. P., and Craige, E.: Echocardiographic studies of the mitral valve in patients with congestive cardiomyopathy and mitral regurgitation, Am. Heart J. 85:413, 1973.

158. Millward, D. K., McLaurin, L. P., and Craige, E.: Echocardiographic studies to explain opening snaps in presence of nonstenotic mitral valves, Am. J. Cardiol. 31:64, 1973.

159. Millward, D. K., McLaurin, L. P., and Craige, E.: Echocardiographic studies of the mitral valve in patients with congestive cardiomyopathy and mitral regurgitation, Circulation 46(Supp. II):42, 1972.

160. Millward, D. K., Robinson, N. J., and Craige, E.: Dissecting aortic aneurysm diagnosed by echocardiography in a patient with rupture of the aneurysm into the right atrium. Rare cause for continuous murmur, Am. J. Cardiol. 30:427, 1972.

161. Moreyra, E., Klein, J. J., Shimada, H., and Segal, B. L.: Idiopathic hypertrophic subaortic stenosis diagnosed by ultrasound, Am. J. Cardiol. 23:32, 1969.

162. Morganroth, J., Henry, W. L., Maron, B. J., Clark, C. E., and Epstein, S. E.: Echocardiographic evidence against idiopathic left ventricular hypertrophy, N. Engl. J. Med. 290:1047, 1974.

163. Moss, A. J., and Adams, F. H. (eds.): *Heart Disease in Infants, Children and Adolescents* (Baltimore: The Williams & Wilkins Company, 1968).

164. Moss, A. J., and Bruhn, F.: The echocardiogram—an ultrasound technique for the detection of pericardial effusion, N. Engl. J. Med. 274: 380, 1966.

165. Nanda, N. C., Gramiak, R., Manning, J., Lipchik, E. O., Mahoney, E. B., and DeWeese, J. A.: Echocardiographic recognition of congenital bicuspid aortic valve, Am. J. Cardiol. 33:159, 1974.

166. Nanda, N. C., Gramiak, R., and Shah, P. M.: Diagnosis of aortic root dissection by echocardiography, Circulation 48:506, 1973.

167. Nanda, N. C., Gramiak, R., Shah, P. M., Chung, K. J., and Robinson, T.: Echocardiographic diagnosis of pulmonary hypertension, Excerpta Medica, International Congress Series, #277, Second World Congress on Ultrasonics in Medicine, Rotterdam, June 4–8, 1973.

168. Nanda, N. C., Gramiak, R., Shah, P. M., DeWeese, J. A., and Mahoney, E. B.: Echocardiographic assessment of left ventricular outflow width in the selection of mitral valve prosthesis, Circulation 48:1208, 1973.

169. Nanda, N. C., Gramiak, R., Shah, P. M., and Lipchik, E. O.: Ultrasound evaluation of mitral valve calcification, Circulation 46(Supp. II): 20, 1972.

170. Neufeld, H. N.: In Moss, A. J., and Adams, F. H. (eds.), *Heart Disease in Infants, Children and Adolescents* (Baltimore: The Williams & Wilkins Company, 1968).

171. Neufeld, H. N., Lucas, R. V., Jr., Lester, R. G., Adams, P., Jr., Anderson, R. C., and Edwards, J. E.: Origin of both great vessels from the right ventricle without pulmonary stenosis, Br. Heart J. 24:393, 1962.

172. Olivia, P. B., Johnson, M. L., Pomerantz, M., and Levene, A.: Dysfunction of the Beall mitral prosthesis and its detection by cinefluoroscope and echocardiography, Am. J. Cardiol. 31:393, 1973.

173. Paraskos, J. A., Grossman, W., Saltz, S., Dalen, J. E., and Dexter, L.: A noninvasive technique for the determination of velocity of circumferential fiber shortening in man, Circ. Res. 29:610, 1971.

174. Pate, J. W., Gardner, H. C., and Norman, R. S.: Diagnosis of pericardial effusion by echocardiography, Ann. Surg. 165:826, 1967.

175. Pfeifer, J., Goldschlager, N., Sweatman, T., Gerbode, E., and Selzer, A.: Malfunction of mitral ball valve prosthesis due to thrombus, Am. J. Cardiol. 29:95, 1972.

176. Pieroni, D. R., Freedom, R. M., and Homcy, E.: Echocardiography in atrio-ventricular canal defects: A clinical spectrum, Excerpta Medica, International Congress Series, Second World Congress on Ultrasonics in Medicine, #277, Rotterdam, June 4–8, 1973, abstract 28, p. 12.

177. Pombo, J. F., Troy, B. L., and Russell, R. O.: Left ventricular volumes and ejection fraction by echocardiography, Circulation 43:480, 1971.

178. Popp, R. L., Brown, O. R., and Harrison, D. C.: Diagnostic accuracy of an ultrasonic multitransducer cardiac imaging system, Circulation 48 (Supp. IV):125, 1973.

179. Popp, R. L., Brown, O. R., Silverman, J., and Harrison, D. C.: Diagnostic use of cardiac echography in the mitral valve prolapse syndromes, Circulation 46 (Supp. II):43, 1972.

180. Popp, R. L., Brown, O. R., Silverman, J. F., and Harrison, D. C.: Echocardiographic abnormalities in the mitral valve prolapse syndrome, Circulation 49:428, 1974.

181. Popp, R. L., and Carmichael, B. M.: Cardiac echography in the diagnosis of prosthetic mitral valve malfunction, Circulation 44(Supp.II):33, 1971.

182. Popp, R. L., and Harrison, D. C.: Ultrasonic cardiac echography for determining stroke volume and valvular regurgitation, Circulation 41: 493, 1970.

183. Popp, R. L., and Harrison, D. C.: Ultrasound in the diagnosis and evaluation of therapy of idiopathic hypertrophic subaortic stenosis, Circulation 40:905, 1969.

184. Popp, R. L., and Harrison, D. C.: Ultrasound for the diagnosis of atrial tumor, Ann. Intern. Med. 71:785, 1969.

185. Popp, R. L., Silverman, J. F., French, J. W., Stinson, E. B., and Harri-

son, D. C.: Echocardiographic findings in discrete subvalvular aortic stenosis, Circulation 49:226, 1974.

186. Popp, R. L., Wolfe, S. B., Hirata, T., and Feigenbaum, H.: Estimation of right and left ventricular size by ultrasound, Am. J. Cardiol. 24:523, 1969.

187. Prakash, R., Atassi, A., Poske, R., and Rosen, K. M.: Prevalence of pericardial effusion and mitral valve involvement in patients with rheumatoid arthritis without cardiac symptoms, N. Engl. J. Med. 289:597, 1973.

188. Pridie, R. B.: Applications of pulse-echo ultrasonics in cardiological diagnosis. Proceedings of the British Institute of Radiology. Abstract printed in Br. J. Radiol. 44:561, 1971.

189. Pridie, R. B., Behnam, R., and Wild, J.: Ultrasound in cardiac diagnosis, Clin. Radiol. 23:160, 1972.

190. Pridie, R. B., Behnam, R., and Oakley, C. M.: Echocardiography of the mitral valve in aortic valve disease, Br. Heart J. 33:296, 1971.

191. Pridie, R. B., and Oakley, C. M.: Mitral valve movement in hypertrophic obstructive cardiomyopathy, Br. Heart J. 31:390, 1969.

192. Quinones, M. A., Gaasch, W. H., Waisser, E., and Alexander, J. K.: Reductions in the rate of diastolic descent of the mitral valve echogram in patients with altered left ventricular diastolic pressure-volume relations, Circulation 49:246, 1974.

193. Roelandt, J., Kloster, F. E., ten Cate, F. J., van Dorp, W. G., Honkoop, J., Bom, N., and Hugenholtz, P. G.: Multidimensional echocardiography. An appraisal of the clinical usefulness, Br. Heart J. 36:29, 1974.

194. Rothman, J., Chase, N. E., Kricheff, I. I., Mayoral, R., and Beranbaum, E. R.: Ultrasonic diagnosis of pericardial effusion, Circulation 35:358, 1967.

195. Sahn, D. J., Deely, W. J., Hagan, A. D., and Friedman, W. F.: Echocardiographic assessment of left ventricular performance in normal newborns, Circulation 49:232, 1974.

196. Sahn, D. J., Terry, R., O'Rourke, R., Leopold, G., and Friedman, W. F.: Multiple crystal echocardiographic evaluation of endocardial cushion defect, Circulation 50:25, 1974.

197. Sahn, D. J., Terry, R., O'Rourke, R., and Friedman, W. F.: Multiple crystal cross-sectional echocardiography in the diagnosis of cyanotic congenital heart disease, Circulation 50:230, 1974.

198. Sahn, D. J., Terry, R., Shackleton, S., and Friedman, W. F.: Validity of structure identification for multicrystal echocardiography, Am. J. Cardiol. 33:167, 1974.

199. Schattenberg, T. T.: Echocardiographic diagnosis of left atrial myxoma, Mayo Clin. Proc. 43:620, 1968.

200. Schelbert, H. R., and Muller, O. F.: Detection of fungal vegetations involving a Starr-Edwards mitral prosthesis by means of ultrasound, Vasc. Surg. 6:20, 1972.

201. Segal, B. L. (guest ed.): Symposium on echocardiography. Diagnostic ultrasound, Am. J. Cardiol. 19:1, 1967.

202. Segal, B. L., Likoff, W., and Kingsley, B.: Echocardiography. Clinical application in mitral stenosis, JAMA 195:99, 1966.

203. Segal, B. L., Likoff, W., and Kingsley, B.: Echocardiography. Clinical application in mitral regurgitation, Am. J. Cardiol. 19:50, 1967.

204. Shah, P. M., Gramiak, R., Adelman, A. G., and Wigle, E. D.: Role of

echocardiography in diagnostic and hemodynamic assessment of hypertrophic subaortic stenosis, Circulation 44:891, 1971.

205. Shah, P. M., Gramiak, R., and Kramer, D. H.: Ultrasound localization of left ventricular outflow obstruction in hypertrophic obstructive cardiomyopathy, Circulation 40:3, 1969.

206. Siggers, D. C., Srivongse, S. A., and Deuchar, D.: Analysis of dynamics of mitral Starr-Edwards valve prosthesis using reflected ultrasound, Br. Heart J. 33:401, 1971.

207. Siggers, D. C., Sivaporn, A., and Srivongse, S. A.: Analysis of dynamics of mitral Starr-Edwards valve prosthesis using reflected ultrasound, Br. Heart J. 32:552, 1970.

208. Sinha, S. N., Hoeschen, R. J., and Miller, A.: Diagnosis of left atrial myxoma by echocardiography, Radiology 108:735, 1973.

209. Sjögren, A. L., Hytönen, I., and Frick, M. H.: Ultrasonic measurements of left ventricular wall thickness, Chest 57:37, 1970.

210. Smyth, M. G., Jr.: In Grossman, C. C., Holmes, J. H., Joyner, C., and Purnell, E. W. (eds.), *Diagnostic Ultrasound. Proceedings of the First International Conference,* University of Pittsburgh, 1965 (New York: Plenum Press, 1966).

211. Solinger, R., Elbl, F., and Minhas, K.: Echocardiography in congenital heart disease, Lancet 2:1093, 1971.

212. Solinger, R., Elbl, F., and Minhas, K.: Echocardiography in the normal neonate, Circulation 47:108, 1973.

213. Solinger, R., Elbl, F., and Minhas, K.: Echocardiographic features of the hypoplastic atrioventricular valve, Circulation 46(Supp. II):224, 1972.

214. Soulen, R. L., Lapayowker, M. S., and Gimenez, J. L.: Echocardiography in the diagnosis of pericardial effusion, Radiology 86:1047, 1966.

215. Sweatman, T., Selzer, A., Kamagaki, M., and Cohn, K.: Echocardiographic diagnosis of mitral regurgitation due to ruptured chordae tendineae, Circulation 46:580, 1972.

216. Sweet, R. L., Russell, R. O., Jr., Moraski, R. E., and Rackley, C. E.: Comparison of left ventricular volumes obtained by biplane angiography and echocardiography in patients with abnormally contracting segments, Circulation 48 (Supp. IV):116, 1973.

217. Tajik, A. J., Gau, G. T., Guiliani, E. R., Ritter, D. G., and Schattenberg, T. T.: Echocardiogram in Ebstein's anomaly with pre-excitation syndrome, type B, Circulation 47:813, 1973.

218. Tajik, A. J., Gau, G. T., Ritter, D. G., and Schattenberg, T. T.: The echocardiographic pattern of right ventricular volume overload in children, Circulation 46(Supp. II):228, 1972.

219. Tajik, A. J., Gau, G. T., Ritter, D. G., and Schattenberg, T. T.: Echocardiographic pattern of right ventricular diastolic volume overload in children, Circulation 46:36, 1972.

220. Tajik, A. J., Gau, G. T., Ritter, D. G., and Schattenberg, T. T.: Illustrative echocardiogram. Echocardiogram in tetralogy of Fallot, Chest 64:107, 1973.

221. Tajik, A. J., Gau, G. T., and Schattenberg, T. T.: Echocardiogram in atrial septal defect, Chest 62:213, 1972.

222. Tajik, A. J., Gau, G. T., and Schattenberg, T. T.: Echocardiographic

"pseudo-IHSS" pattern in atrial septal defect, Chest 62:324, 1972.

223. Tajik, A. J., Gau, G. T., Schattenberg, T. T., and Ritter, D. G.: Normal ventricular septal motion in atrial septal defect, Mayo Clin. Proc. 47: 635, 1972.

224. Tajik, A. J., Gau, G. T., and Schattenberg, T. T.: Echocardiogram in total anomalous pulmonary venous drainage, Mayo Clin. Proc. 47:247, 1972.

225. Ting, Y. M.: Ultrasound cardiography in diagnosis of mitral insufficiency, Radiology 109:253, 1973.

226. Troy, B. L., Pombo, J., and Rackley, C. E.: Measurement of left ventricular wall thickness and mass by echocardiography, Circulation 45:602, 1972.

227. Ultan, L. B., Segal, B. L., and Likoff, W.: Echocardiography in congenital heart disease, Am. J. Cardiol. 19:74, 1967.

228. Van Dorp, W. G., Kloster, F. E., ten Cate, F. J., Paladino, D., Roelandt, J., and Bom, N.: The spectrum of mitral valve motion seen by multiple element echocardiography (multiscan), Circulation 48 (Supp. IV):226, 1973.

229. Walter, C. (ed.): *Electrical Hazards in Hospitals. Proceedings of a Workshop* (Washington, D.C.: National Academy of Sciences, 1970).

230. Warshawsky, J. K., Neal, W. A., Allen, H. D., Blieden, L., Lucas, R. V., Jr., and Warwick, W. J.: Echocardiography in cystic fibrosis. Presented at the Cystic Fibrosis Club, National Cystic Fibrosis Research Foundation, Washington, D.C., 1974.

231. Watts, L. E., Barnes, R. W., and Nomeir, A. M.: Ultrasound evaluation of mitral valve prostheses, Excerpta Medica, International Congress Series, #277, Second World Congress on Ultrasonics in Medicine, Rotterdam, #30, p. 14, June 4–8, 1973.

232. Wells, P. N.: *Physical Principles of Ultrasonic Diagnosis* (London and New York: Academic Press, 1969).

233. Weyman, A. E., Dillon, J. C., Feigenbaum, H., and Chang, S.: Echocardiographic patterns of pulmonic valve motion in pulmonic stenosis, Am. J. Cardiol. 33:178, 1974.

234. Wharton, C. F. P., and Bescos, L. L.: Mitral valve movement. A study using an ultrasound technique, Br. Heart J. 32:344, 1970.

235. Williams, R. G., and Rudd, M.: Echocardiographic features of endocardial cushion defects, Circulation 49:418, 1974.

236. Winsberg, F.: Rapid systolic oscillations of the aortic valve. A normal finding, Excerpta Medica, International Congress Series, #277, Second World Congress on Ultrasonics in Medicine, Rotterdam, June 4–8, 1973.

237. Winsberg, F., Gabor, G. E., Hernberg, J. G., and Weiss, B.: Fluttering of the mitral valve in aortic insufficiency, Circulation 41:225, 1970.

238. Winsberg, F., and Mercer, E. N.: Echocardiography in combined valve disease, Radiology 105:405, 1972.

239. Winsberg, F., Yeh, H-C., and Mercer, E. N.: Echographic aortic valve orifice dimension. Its use in evaluating aortic stenosis and cardiac output, Circulation 48(Supp. IV):231, 1973.

240. Winters, W. L., Gimenez, J., and Soloff, L. A.: Clinical application of ultrasound in the analysis of prosthetic ball valve function, Am. J. Cardiol. 19:97, 1967.

241. Wise, J. R., Cleland, W. P., Hallidie-Smith, K. A., Bentall, H., Goodwin, J. F., and Oakley, C. M.: Urgent aortic valve replacement for acute aortic regurgitation due to infective endocarditis, Br. Heart J. 31:797, 1969.
242. Wolfe, S. B., Popp, R. L., and Feigenbaum, H.: Diagnosis of atrial tumors by ultrasound, Circulation 39:615, 1969.
243. Womersley, J. R.: An elastic tube theory of pulse transmission and oscillatory flow in mammalian arteries, Wright Air Development Center Technical Report, WADC-TR 56-614, 1957.
244. Woodward, B., and Warwick, R.: How safe is diagnostic sonar?, Br. J. Radiol. 43:719, 1970.
245. Yuste, P., Aza, V., Mingues, I., Cerezo, L., and Martinez-Bordiu, C.: Dissecting aortic aneurysm diagnosed by echocardiography. A pre- and postoperative study, Br. Heart J. 36:111, 1974.

Index

319